The Social Determinants of Mental Health

The Social Determinants of Mental Health

Edited by

Michael T. Compton, M.D., M.P.H.
Ruth S. Shim, M.D., M.P.H.

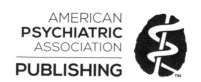

AMERICAN
PSYCHIATRIC
ASSOCIATION
PUBLISHING

If you would like to buy between 25 and 99 copies of this or any other American Psychiatric Publishing title, you are eligible for a 20% discount; please contact Customer Service at appi@psych.org or 800-368-5777. If you wish to buy 100 or more copies of the same title, please e-mail us at bulksales@psych.org for a price quote.

Copyright © 2015 American Psychiatric Association
ALL RIGHTS RESERVED

Manufactured in the United States of America on acid-free paper
18   17   5   4   3
First Edition

Typeset in Swis721 Md BT and Palatino Lt Std

American Psychiatric Publishing
A Division of American Psychiatric Association
1000 Wilson Boulevard
Arlington, VA 22209-3901
www.appi.org

Library of Congress Cataloging-in-Publication Data
The social determinants of mental health / edited by Michael T. Compton, Ruth S. Shim.—First edition.

  p. ; cm.

Includes bibliographical references and index.

ISBN 978-1-58562-477-5 (pb : alk. paper)

I. Compton, Michael T., editor. II. Shim, Ruth S., 1977– , editor. III. American Psychiatric Publishing, publisher.

[DNLM: 1. Mental Health—United States. 2. Socioeconomic Factors—United States. WM 31]

RC455

362.19689dc23

2014039125

British Library Cataloguing in Publication Data
A CIP record is available from the British Library.

Contents

The Group for the Advancement of Psychiatry (GAP)
Prevention Committee
Ruth S. Shim, M.D., M.P.H.
Michael T. Compton, M.D., M.P.H.
Marc W. Manseau, M.D., M.P.H.
Carol Koplan, M.D.
Frederick J.P. Langheim, M.D., Ph.D.
Rebecca A. Powers, M.D., M.P.H.

Jane A. Rafferty, M.A.
Jamie M. Abelson, M.S.W.
Kimson Bryant, B.A.
James S. Jackson, Ph.D.

Carol Koplan, M.D.
Anna Chard, M.P.H.

Contributors

Jamie M. Abelson, M.S.W.
Senior Research Associate, Institute for Social Research, University of Michigan, Ann Arbor

Kimson Bryant, B.A.
Research Associate, Institute for Social Research, University of Michigan, Ann Arbor, Michigan

Earle Chambers, Ph.D., M.P.H.
Assistant Professor, Department of Family and Social Medicine, Albert Einstein College of Medicine, Bronx, New York

Anna Chard, M.P.H.
Public Health Program Associate, Department of Environmental Health, Rollins School of Public Health, Emory University, Atlanta, Georgia

Michael T. Compton, M.D., M.P.H.
Chairman, Department of Psychiatry, Lenox Hill Hospital; Professor, Department of Psychiatry, Hofstra North Shore LIJ School of Medicine at Hofstra University, New York, New York

Benjamin G. Druss, M.D., M.P.H.
Professor and Rosalynn Carter Chair, Department of Health Policy and Management, Rollins School of Public Health, Emory University, Atlanta, Georgia

Kisha B. Holden, Ph.D., M.S.C.R.
Associate Professor, Department of Psychiatry and Behavioral Sciences, Morehouse School of Medicine, Atlanta, Georgia

Christopher S. Holliday, Ph.D., M.A., M.P.H.
Director, Population Health, Improving Health Outcomes, American Medical Association, Chicago, Illinois

James S. Jackson, Ph.D.
Director and Research Professor, Institute for Social Research, Daniel Katz Distinguished University Professor of Psychology, University of Michigan, Ann Arbor, Michigan

Carol Koplan, M.D.
Adjunct Assistant Professor, Department of Behavioral Sciences and Health Education, Rollins School of Public Health, Emory University, Atlanta, Georgia

Frederick J.P. Langheim, M.D., Ph.D.
Medical Director of Consultation and Liaison Psychiatry, St. Mary's Hospital; Staff Psychiatrist, Dean Health System; Clinical Adjunct Assistant Professor, University of Wisconsin–Madison, Madison, Wisconsin

Marc W. Manseau, M.D., M.P.H.
Clinical Assistant Professor, Department of Psychiatry, New York University School of Medicine, New York, New York

Sir Michael Marmot, M.B.B.S., M.P.H., Ph.D.
Director, Institute of Health Equity; Professor, Department of Epidemiology and Public Health, University College London, London, UK

Brian S. McGregor, Ph.D.
Instructor, Department of Psychiatry and Behavioral Sciences, Morehouse School of Medicine, Atlanta, Georgia

Rebecca A. Powers, M.D., M.P.H.
Associate Professor, Adjunct Clinical Faculty, Department of Psychiatry and Behavioral Sciences, Stanford University School of Medicine, Stanford, California

Jane A. Rafferty, M.A.
Senior Research Associate, Institute for Social Research, University of Michigan, Ann Arbor, Michigan

Megan T. Sandel, M.D., M.P.H.
Associate Professor, Department of Pediatrics, Boston University Schools of Medicine and Public Health, Boston, Massachusetts

David Satcher, M.D., Ph.D.
Director, Satcher Health Leadership Institute; Poussaint-Satcher-Cosby Chair in Mental Health, Morehouse School of Medicine, Atlanta, Georgia

Ruth S. Shim, M.D., M.P.H.
Vice Chair, Education and Faculty Development, Department of Psychiatry, Lenox Hill Hospital; Associate Professor, Department of Psychiatry, Hofstra North Shore–LIJ School of Medicine at Hofstra University, New York, New York

Shakira F. Suglia, Sc.D., M.S.
Assistant Professor, Department of Epidemiology, Mailman School of Public Health, Columbia University, New York, New York

Lynn C. Todman, Ph.D., M.C.P.
Research Affiliate, Community Innovators Laboratory, Massachusetts Institute of Technology, Cambridge, Massachusetts

Disclosure of Interests

The contributors to this book have indicated that they have no financial inter-ests or other affiliations that represent or could appear to represent a competing interest with their contributions to this book.

The Social Determinants of Mental Health: From Evidence to Policy

Mental illness has been the dark secret of families and societies. For an individual to admit to it incurred public shame. Being mentally ill shaded into being morally lacking. For the medical profession it was the nonserious end of practice—no fancy diagnostic techniques, no heroic treatments. For a set of conditions that will affect a third or more of people at some point in their lives, this neglect is quite remarkable...and shameful.

At long last there are moves afoot to redress this neglect. There is a long way to go, but there are glimmers of recognition that more should be done on diagnosis and treatment and that discrimination against people with mental illness is indefensible. This book addresses a third important issue: the social determinants of mental health and illness. It is timely and welcome.

Those of us concerned with social determinants of health and health equity cannot ignore mental illness because it is such an important effect, for good and ill, of how we organize our affairs in society. Those concerned primarily with mental illness cannot ignore social determinants because therein lies the prospect of improving mental health and preventing mental illness. This book is enormously helpful in showing the pathways from social norms and public policies to mental illness. It emphasizes the life course—harmful effects on adult mental illness begin with adverse early life experiences—and shows how social determinants can lead to stress with consequent psychological and physiological pathways to disease and to poor choices and risky behaviors. A key insight is that the same set of causal pathways from society to the individual can have adverse effects on both mental and physical illness.

In some quarters it is almost a reflex, which involves little cerebral activity, to blame poor people for their poor behavior and bad health.

Demonstrating, as this book does, how the social environment constrains choices and behaviors suggests that such a reflex is not based on an understanding of the scientific evidence.

A theme of the book is that understanding of the importance of social determinants of health has grown in many countries but has had little penetration of the policy process in the United States. If the book, in addition to its impressive bringing together of the scientific evidence on social determinants of mental health, succeeds in influencing U.S. policies and social norms, it will have done us all a wonderful service.

Sir Michael Marmot, M.B.B.S, M.P.H., Ph.D.

Preface

The basic premise of this book is that society plays a prominent role in creating and shaping poor mental health and mental illnesses. As such, society is also in a position to improve mental health and reduce risk for mental illnesses.

Where an individual, a family, a community, or a society is located on the continuum from health and wellness to illness and infirmity is multi-determined. Genetic influences and biological constitution are undoubtedly key drivers of health and wellness, but the contexts of the individual, family, community, and society are also crucial. In this book, we focus on those social and environmental contexts. At an even deeper level, we focus on society, specifically, America in the twenty-first century.

We begin with an in-depth overview in Chapter 1, which shows how an *unwell society* (one with *public policies* and *social norms* that, left unimproved, will continue to drive poor mental health) and an *unfair society* (one characterized by prominent inequalities in the distribution of opportunity) undergird the diverse social determinants of poor mental health and behavioral disorders. In Chapters 2–10 we then articulate how such factors as racial discrimination, adverse early life experiences, unemployment and underemployment, and poor access to health care, to name a few, have an impact on risk for and outcomes of mental illnesses. Although such *social determinants of health,* or *fundamental causes,* or *causes of the causes,* might appear to be quite far upstream compared with the more proximal risk factors that they create, they set the stage for poor mental health, and indeed mental illnesses, including substance use disorders, in individuals and communities. Note that in using the word *social,* we refer to both interactions among people and interactions between people and their surroundings. As such, how society distributes education, jobs, wealth, food, and housing is *social,* as are the health care system and policies pertaining to it. We outline (for psychiatrists and other mental health professionals primarily but for diverse other audiences as well) some of the many ways in which society *creates* and *sustains* poor mental health and, indeed, diagnosed or diagnosable mental illnesses, including substance use disorders. Some of the clinical vignettes in Chapters 2–10 pertain to persons with serious mental illnesses because psychiatrists represent one of our intended audiences, but in such instances, the story would be just as relevant if it referred to milder poor mental health and related outcomes. In pointing out society's role in poor mental health outcomes, we also begin to show how society (i.e., all of us) can create mental *health* and *resilience*. In Chapter 11 we encourage everyone to take action and suggest ways to start doing so.

Unlike addressing the biological determinants of health and disease (e.g., genetics), addressing the social determinants of mental health inherently involves policy and politics. We have no a priori political agenda, but political considerations cannot be avoided if we are to adequately consider this topic and make progress in this arena. Mental health and risk for mental illnesses are substantially shaped by policy and politics, and taking action to promote mental health and reduce risk for mental illnesses is thus a political and policy-related process. For example, a youth's quality and extent of education certainly have long-term health implications, and improving educational quality, reducing high school dropout, and enhancing access to higher education for all are objectives that clearly necessitate a policy and political approach. Enacting policy requires discussion and compromise that evoke one's own political perspectives as well as those of the groups to which one belongs.

We are not policy makers or politicians, however. We are psychiatrists. We are extensively experienced in evaluating patients, diagnosing mental illnesses and substance use disorders, and developing plans and programs for optimal treatment. In designing, compiling, and editing this book, we have turned our attention from patients to communities and, more broadly, from communities to society. We have "evaluated" our society with regard to its role in creating risk for poor mental health. From this assessment, we have arrived at the "diagnosis" that our society is in some respects unwell and in many ways unfair. As a result, we have begun a process (which undoubtedly will need to be set forth in greater detail elsewhere) of developing plans for optimal "treatment" for society to become well and fair.

Because we are psychiatrists, our primary audience will most likely be mental health professionals. For this reason, in this book we repeatedly refer to psychiatrists and other mental health professionals and provide clinical vignettes involving patients to illuminate concepts at both the population and individual patient levels. In fact, our greatest dilemma in preparing this book has been the difficult task of trying to balance the individual/clinical/patient perspectives and the population/public health/community points of view. However, ultimately addressing and treating the problems that we point out will require society (i.e., all of us) to work in a unified, willful, and health-smart way. Clinicians can take certain actions, but the real solution to reducing risk for mental illnesses and optimizing mental health depends on political will, advocacy, and collective action in which we *all* participate.

Having briefly introduced the content of the book, we will now tell you a bit about ourselves. How did we arrive at diagnosing unhealthy public policies and social norms and unequal distribution of opportunity within society as the societal "disorders" of primary interest to us within the field of psychiatry? It was largely an unplanned and uncharted journey. Choosing psychiatry as a medical specialty was itself a personal journey for both of us, one that is beyond the purview of this brief preface. Our shared journey, however, began on completion of our psychiatry training. Somewhat disillusioned by the limited effectiveness of psychiatric treatments—and impressed by the fact that many of our patients (especially those whom we evaluated and treated at Grady Health System in downtown Atlanta) struggle with social problems that often overshadow their mental illness—we both completed a fellowship in community psychiatry and public health. This 2-year experience and master of public health degree prepared us to embrace a population-based, public health framework that would come to complement our patient-based, medical/psychiatric perspective. As such, concepts such as prevention, health promotion, and social justice became as important to us as treatment and standard psychiatric care.

A number of years after our community psychiatry and public health fellowship training, we found ourselves amid a small group of like-minded colleagues in the Prevention Committee of an organization called the Group for the Advancement of Psychiatry (GAP). Many discussions within this committee (whose members wrote Chapter 1, with individual committee members also writing several other chapters) gravitated toward issues pertaining to health disparities and inequities and other social injustices. In our work to promote prevention within the field of psychiatry, we often found ourselves discussing policy approaches rather than clinical ones. The committee decided—after vigorous thinking around the table; sharing ideas at breakfast, lunch, and dinner at the GAP meeting each April and November; and debates and discussions at the juice bar—that moving toward genuine prevention in psychiatry would require digging deeper than the proximal risk factors;

we would have to look toward the causes of the causes, or the fundamental causes. Furthermore, for prevention of mental illnesses and promotion of mental health for all, we would have to look at those factors in our society that drive the causes of the causes. This decision led us to focus not only on the set of *core* social determinants of mental health (e.g., unemployment, food insecurity, housing instability) outlined in Chapters 2–10 but also on two substrata from which these core social determinants derive: an unfair society (because of the unequal distribution of opportunity) and an unwell society (by virtue of public policies that require health-focused optimization and social norms that must be shifted to achieve health). This shared journey resulted in the book that you are about to discover.

Having briefly introduced ourselves and the inspiration for this line of inquiry, we will now tell you more about the book itself. Following the overview (Chapter 1), which lays out our guiding principles and our framework in greater detail, the authors of Chapters 2–10 elaborate on discrimination and social exclusion; adverse early life experiences; poor education; unemployment, underemployment, and job insecurity; income inequality, poverty, and neighborhood deprivation; food insecurity; poor housing quality and housing instability; adverse features of the built environment; and poor access to health care as core social determinants of mental health. As noted earlier, Chapter 11 urges us all to take action. We settled on this way of organizing the book because it allows us to focus on one social determinant at a time. Other structures could have been used; for example, a life course approach or developmental perspective would have been equally informative, outlining social determinants and how they affect children, adolescents, adults, and older adults and the elderly.

In describing the structure of the book, we should take a moment to specifically thank two special contributors. Both have immeasurably shaped the field of public health and fearlessly challenged us all to do more to address the social determinants of mental health. First, Sir Michael Marmot, who provided the thoughtful foreword, "The Social Determinants of Mental Health: From Evidence to Policy," is the world's leader and foremost expert on the social determinants of health. He has worked tirelessly to advance the science and implore societies to take action to address the social determinants of health and has achieved significant results in the process. Second, it is only fitting that Dr. David Satcher, the 16th surgeon general of the United States, has the final word in this book as a coauthor of the last chapter, which is a call to action. Beginning in 1999 with the publication of *Mental Health: A Report of the*

Surgeon General and building on this work with the 2001 supplement, *Mental Health: Culture, Race, and Ethnicity,* Dr. Satcher has unwaveringly advocated for improving mental health diagnosis and treatment and addressing disparities and inequities in health in ways that no other governmental figure has done before or since.

We would like to point out a number of particularities about this book. First, although a relatively simple semantic issue, the terminology *social determinants of health* is imprecise in that the factors commonly called social determinants of *health* (e.g., adverse early life experiences, income inequality) are actually social determinants of *poor* health and *illnesses.* We will follow the commonly used terminology and refer to the *social determinants of mental health* even though these determinants lead to risk for poor mental health and mental illnesses.

Second, again with regard to semantics, the term *social determinants of mental health* emphasizes *mental,* although these determinants are related to diverse physical, psychiatric, behavioral, and social outcomes. They are also linked to the various substance use disorders. As such, the *mental* terminology is shorthand for diverse psychological, social, and behavioral outcomes. At times, we use *behavioral health* or *behavioral disorders,* the latter indicating mental illnesses and substance use disorders as a combined group.

Third, we focus on the United States, even though the topic is of great relevance across the globe and perhaps has even greater pertinence in low- and middle-income countries than in the United States. Several societies have made significant strides in addressing the social determinants of health, as evidenced by advances in Canada, the United Kingdom, the Scandinavian countries, and Australia. The United States lags behind in terms of implementing effective interventions to address the social determinants of health. This lag stems from a cultural perspective that is quite unique when compared with that of other countries. In the United States, policy change often requires striking a delicate balance between protecting and promoting the collective health of the population on the one hand and preserving autonomy and the individual freedoms of citizens on the other. It is our intention to consider and learn from the progress made in other countries and to begin to assemble the evidence to support taking action on these issues in the United States.

Fourth, another particularity of this book is that we artificially isolate social determinants from genetic and other biological determinants of health and disease, even though they clearly interact with one another and are actually linked in many ways. The biopsychosocial model that many psychiatrists are exposed to in training emphasizes this interaction. The environment changes our genes (in diverse ways, including epigenetics), and our genes change the environment (because they give rise to us all and we are continuously changing the environment around us). Most chronic medical conditions, including most psychiatric illnesses, are currently conceptualized as having a multitude of genetic, behavioral, and social determinants. We isolate the social determinants just to allow for a concise overview of existing knowledge and a clear set of directions that clinicians, policy makers, and others can take. It is also artificial to separate mental health from physical health and the social determinants of mental health from the social determinants of physical health. The social determinants of mental health are largely the same as those underpinning chronic physical health conditions (e.g., diabetes, hypertension, cardiovascular disease, cancer). We specifically delineate the social determinants of mental health in order to translate the existing body of literature to the mental health arena, again allowing for articulation of specific actions that clinicians, policy makers, and others can take.

Fifth, we recognize that we have not considered all of the social determinants that exist, either in the United States or globally. Some social determinants that should be considered but are not addressed include transportation limitations; exposure to natural disasters and other large-scale stressful events; global warming and climate change; and exposure to war, gun violence, and trauma in adulthood. Additionally, we acknowledge that most of the selected social determinants of mental health presented in Chapters 2–10 are closely linked to social isolation, social exclusion, and inequities and injustices; these topics are so important that entire books would be needed to lay out their significance to health. We also have not covered classism, sexism, or homophobia, which obviously also contribute to social exclusion, inequities, and injustices. We recognize these limitations while aspiring to give readers a general overview of an expansive topic in a single volume that is not intimidatingly lengthy.

Sixth, for the purposes of clarity and concision, the social determinants have been artificially segregated from one another. We readily acknowledge that most of the social determinants of mental health are intricately linked to one another. They rarely occur in isolation, and individuals, communities, or societies affected by one are typically affected by many, if not most, others. Just as the social determinants co-occur, the adverse outcomes that they predict and provoke co-occur. Thus, although at times we comment separately on specific physical health conditions (e.g., obesity, diabetes, cardiovascular disease) and specific behavioral disorders (e.g., mood disorders, anxiety disorders, substance use disorders), these illnesses are highly comorbid. Individuals affected by one are more likely to be affected by the others. As such, some individuals are affected by multiple social determinants and risk factors, as well as by multiple adverse outcomes. As a parallel to the fact that some individuals are disproportionately affected by social determinants and adverse outcomes, the same is true of some population groups. For example, African Americans as a group continue to be unfairly and disparately affected by the social determinants detailed throughout this book. The same is true of native/indigenous groups and tribal communities.

Seventh, to make them easier to discuss, we often treat the social determinants as categorical (e.g., employment vs. unemployment, stable housing vs. housing instability). In reality, they each exist on a continuum rather than being categorical phenomena. For example, we all have some level of exposure to adverse early life experiences, and we all contend with adverse features of the built environment around us to a variable extent. Categorizing simply makes for easier writing and reading, although the social determinants are undoubtedly dimensional constructs.

Eighth, although numerous *social risk factors* have been identified and are familiar to mental health professionals, we focus instead on the more far-reaching and pervasive social determinants that have clear policy implications. For example, being unmarried, living alone, and having had a family member who committed suicide are commonly cited social risk factors for suicide, and a more urban upbringing, cannabis use in adolescence, and declining social functioning in adolescence are widely known as some of the social risk factors for schizophrenia; however, such individual level, proximal social risk factors are not addressed in this book. We focus instead on the broader, deeper social factors affecting society as a whole and those with clear policy implications.

Our ultimate goal with this book is to increase knowledge about the potential for policy change and the shifting of social norms to address poor mental health and mental illnesses in the United States. We all have the power to act in the creating of a culture of positive mental health and wellness, in which children are born into secure and stable environments, grow up in settings free from trauma and other adverse early life experiences, receive high-quality and equal education and nurturing social support, and have endless and equal opportunities for success and fulfillment throughout their lives. The call to action aspect of this book is complex in that there is not a single action but a multitude of possible actions that must go hand in hand. To find a place to begin taking action, we recommend that each reader carefully consider the diversity of topics presented and then select an action or series of actions on the basis of his or her own particular interests and passions. For some, that might mean volunteering in a parenting skills program; for others it might mean working to bring a farmers' market to a disenfranchised neighborhood; and for others it might mean serving on the board of a local housing and urban planning agency. None of us can do it all, but all of us can do something.

Michael T. Compton, M.D., M.P.H.
Ruth S. Shim, M.D., M.P.H.

Acknowledgments

The writing or editing of any book is a collaborative effort, and acknowledgments are often extensive. To be brief, we thank John McDuffie, Rebecca Rinehart, and Robert E. Hales, M.D., M.B.A., at American Psychiatric Publishing for their remarkable support of this project. We ask forgiveness from all the chapter authors for our seemingly countless e-mails with deadlines; the end product of your work is, indeed, beautiful. We honor our patients over the years, whose difficulties pointed us to what we see as the real issues pertaining to mental health and mental illnesses. We thank countless colleagues, employees, bosses, friends, and loved ones who were patient as we often seemed distracted by the work of compiling this book. Most importantly, we offer gratitude to Carol, Becca, Fred, and Marc; they empowered us and entrusted us with the role of editors to put forth our shared ideas.

1

Overview of the Social Determinants of Mental Health

The Group for the Advancement of Psychiatry (GAP) Prevention Committee
Ruth S. Shim, M.D., M.P.H.
Michael T. Compton, M.D., M.P.H.
Marc W. Manseau, M.D., M.P.H.
Carol Koplan, M.D.
Frederick J.P. Langheim, M.D., Ph.D.
Rebecca A. Powers, M.D., M.P.H.

Do we not always find the diseases of the populace traceable to defects in society?

Rudolf Virchow, 1821–1902

Some might say that we live in trying times in the United States. Although many individuals are doing well, even thriving, large segments of the American population deal with the deleterious consequences of high rates of unemployment, poverty, economic inequality, exposure to violence, and other detrimental social experiences. In addition, the prevalence of adverse health behaviors and poor lifestyle choices is alarming, and rates of chronic disease have skyrocketed, with approximately 133 million Americans currently living with at least one chronic illness, a number projected to increase in upcoming years (Wu and Green 2000). Additionally, more people are living with multiple chronic conditions, including both physical and behavioral health disorders. Although genetic underpinnings help explain vulnerability for these chronic health conditions, we cannot ignore the many nongenetic contributions (i.e., those of society and our environment) in the development and persistence of chronic disease.

When considering mental illnesses, the epidemiological facts are particularly concerning. Mental illnesses are highly prevalent, affecting almost half (46.4%) of all Americans at some point in their lifetime (Kessler et al. 2005). Given this high prevalence, one might say we are in the midst of a mental illness epidemic, even if the prevalence is relatively static. Depression is a leading cause of disability and disease burden worldwide (Ferrari et al. 2013). Record numbers of individuals with serious mental illnesses are being treated in jails and prisons, often considered the *de facto* mental health system in America (Torrey 1995). Returning veterans of wars in Iraq (Operation Iraqi Freedom) and Afghanistan (Operation Enduring Freedom) have high rates of posttraumatic stress disorder (PTSD) and suicide (Jakupcak et al. 2009) in addition to traumatic brain injuries and physical disabilities including amputations. PTSD is also on the rise among civilian populations, particularly among individuals living in low-income, urban settings (Breslau et al. 1998; Donley et al. 2012; Reese et al. 2012). Epidemics of gun violence and substance use disorders also contribute to mortality among many vulnerable populations in the United States. For individuals with serious mental illnesses such as bipolar disorder and schizophrenia, a number of factors contribute to limited treatment and poor health outcomes, including life expectancy reduced by up to 25 years on average compared with individuals without such conditions (Parks et al. 2006).

With these sobering statistics, one might feel disheartened about the state of mental illness prevention, diagnosis, and treatment in the United States. However, there are many reasons to be optimistic despite the current landscape. The field of psychiatry has made great strides in the management and treatment of many mental illnesses, including new medications, new evidence that supports the effectiveness of various behavioral therapies and psychosocial treatments, and advances in understanding the genetic architecture of risk for mental illnesses and substance use disorders. Furthermore, many individuals at apparent higher risk for mental illnesses or substance use disorders possess resilience that protects them from developing such conditions. The recovery movement, which promotes hope, empowerment, peer support, and shared decision making, has emphasized that individuals with mental illnesses can live full, productive, and rewarding lives, a goal not always considered possible in the past. Further neurobiological advancements are on the horizon, with committed financial investment in cutting-edge research, including the federal government's Brain Research through Advancing Innovative Neurotechnologies (BRAIN) Initiative (Insel et al. 2013).

Significant progress is certainly being made, yet many challenges still lie ahead. Throughout history, there have been shifts in the balance between emphasis on the social environment versus emphasis on innate biology as the primary cause of disease and disability. This ongoing debate, commonly referred to as *nature versus nurture*, seems to have given way to a mutual understanding within the mental health field. The medical model in mental health care has largely shifted to the biopsychosocial model, and there is a widely held understanding that both nature *and* nurture contribute to the development and persistence of disease. In light of greater recognition of this complex interplay, the fields of medicine and mental health have invested significant resources, funding, and energy in advancing scientific research and discovery around molecular, genetic, and neurobiological breakthroughs in mental health diagnosis and treatment. Unfortunately, however, we have not seen a commensurate dedication to addressing how social and environmental factors contribute to these illnesses or how factors pertaining to society and the environment influence or interact with genetics and neurobiology. In order to effectively prevent and manage mental illnesses, we need to appropriately consider the role that environmental and social factors play in causing and sustaining disease and also to consider the role of political power, policy action, resource distribution, and program development and dissemination in addressing these factors.

In this book we focus on those factors that contribute to health and illness that are addressable through policy and programs, environmental change, and both collective and individual decisions within society; such factors have been most commonly referred to as the *social determinants of health*. Remarkably, these underlying factors tend to be the same for both physical health conditions and mental health conditions. Given our focus on articulating their impact on mental health and mental or behavioral disorders, we refer to them as the *social determinants of mental health*.

Defining the Social Determinants of Health

The World Health Organization defines the social determinants of health as the conditions in which people "are born, grow, live, work, and age" and notes that they are shaped by the multilevel distribution of money, power, and resources (World Health Organization 2008; Centers for Disease Control and Prevention 2014). This perspective places the responsibility of health and health equity firmly within the realms of politics, policies, and governance and encourages lawmakers to consider the health impacts of all policies (World Health Organization 2008). This concept and approach to reducing health inequities is not new. Societies that invest their money, power, and resources in addressing these social determinants of health have been able to improve health outcomes over time. International evidence and success stories are accumulating, but for complex reasons, these findings have been somewhat ignored, or at least slow to gain traction, in the United States (World Health Organization 2012).

Although the social determinants of health are a prominent focus of the field of public health, the technologically oriented, individual treatment–based field of medicine (which includes psychiatry) tends to lose sight of the social determinants. The social determinants of health (e.g., discrimination and social exclusion; adverse early life experiences; poor education; unemployment, underemployment, and job insecurity; income inequality, poverty, and neighborhood deprivation; poor access to sufficient healthy food; poor housing quality and housing instability; adverse features of the built environment; poor access to health care) predispose individuals and populations to poor health. Although they can be dealt with at the individual level (i.e., in the clinic or social services setting), they are most powerfully addressed by improving policies and disseminating effective programs. In this book, we present ways of assessing and addressing the various social determinants of mental health within the United States in the clinical setting while also presenting some ways in which mental health professionals and others can be involved in policy and programmatic solutions to the social determinants.

Defining the Social Determinants of Mental Health

As noted above, the social determinants of mental health are, for the most part, not distinct from the social determinants of physical health and, as such, are not defined differently. As with the general concept of the social determinants of health, the idea of the social determinants of mental health is not new. For example, as early as 1897, Émile Durkheim emphasized the role of the social environment on rates of suicide (Durkheim 1951). Similarly, a rich history within the field of social epidemiology specifically addresses the social determinants of mental health through population-level research.

Despite the lack of major differences between the social determinants of health and the social determinants of mental health, for several reasons, the social determinants of mental health deserve special emphasis. As previously noted, mental illnesses are highly prevalent and highly disabling. Mental illnesses are highly comorbid conditions and are commonly associated with other mental illnesses, substance use disorders, and chronic health conditions, including pulmonary, cardiovascular, and cerebrovascular diseases (Goodell et al. 2011). As a result, mental disorders and substance use disorders, are high-cost illnesses. Costs are both societal and personal and can be measured in terms of health care costs, decreased productivity, absenteeism, and damaged relationships. When considering physical health and the social determinants of health, one cannot ignore the role or impact of mental health.

Although some mental illnesses (such as schizophrenia and bipolar disorder) have substantial heritability (i.e., genetic underpinnings), the onset and course of illness are often influenced by social determinants. Using schizophrenia as an example, the causes of schizophrenia are thought of as component causes, meaning that constellations of individual genetic and socioenvironmental risk factors—those factors that precede the disease and are statistically associated with the disease—differ from one affected person to the next and set the stage for various manifestations of psychosis. In some people, schizophrenia might be strictly genetic, as in 22q11 deletion syndrome; in others, the genetic underpinnings might be overshadowed by an accumulation of environmental (i.e., nongenetic) risk factors. Obviously, for the greatest impact from a prevention perspective at the population level, interventions that address both biological factors and the socioenvironmental landscape may be the most productive. Furthermore, the severity and outcomes of mental illnesses are often affected by social determinants. As a result, major strides can be made not only in prevention of certain mental illnesses but also in treatment and recovery from others. Social and environmental factors have been underemphasized in recent years, presenting opportunities for major breakthroughs in the prevention and treatment of mental illnesses.

Reasons to Address the Social Determinants of Mental Health

We must address the social determinants of mental health for several reasons. First, treatments for some mental illnesses remain very limited, with moderate effects on outcomes at best. Because we are rarely able to cure or fully manage mental illnesses with medical interventions, we need to provide ways for people living with mental illnesses to lead healthy, fulfilling, and meaningful lives, which involves attention to economic, social, and environmental factors. Second, even if we discovered highly effective medical treatments for mental illnesses, we know that such disorders are initially caused by complex interactions between biological, social, and environmental factors. Therefore, paying attention to the social factors—many of which are amenable to public health and policy interventions—will arguably always be necessary for the efficient and cost-effective prevention of mental illnesses on the population level. Finally, and perhaps most importantly, because the social determinants of mental health are largely responsible for inequalities in mental health, attention to the social determinants of mental health is a moral imperative. It is one important way to make society more fair and just, giving everyone an equal opportunity to live a healthy and satisfying life free from mental illnesses and disability.

Key Concepts Relevant to the Social Determinants of Mental Health

Central to the social determinants of mental health approach is shifting the concept of mental illnesses from an individual patient approach to a public health, population-based approach. Public health principles are essential when considering the social determinants of mental health, and in doing so, one must appreciate the role of risk and protective factors, recognize the intergenerational perspective, and attend to social justice and health equity.

Population-Based, Public Health Approach to Mental Health

In 1999, the surgeon general published the first ever report on mental health in the United States (U.S. Department of Health and Human Services 1999), describing the population-based goal of prevention of mental illnesses and promotion of mental health and giving legitimacy to the inclusion of mental health within the field of public health. Public health addresses the health of communities and populations rather than that of only individuals. The public health approach aims to reduce mental disorders and advance mental health through prevention, health promotion, and an emphasis on wellness. The field of public health uses epidemiology and surveillance to determine the age of onset, incidence, and prevalence of disease; these data are used to develop evidence-based programs and interventions to prevent and reduce disorders in at-risk populations. In the study of mental illnesses, epidemiology and surveillance are instrumental in determining where disparities and inequalities in health exist, as well as overall health outcomes and effectiveness of treatment. Also central to this approach is the consideration of population health across the entire life span.

Psychiatrists and other mental health professionals often see poor mental health from the perspective of an individual patient in a medical or psychiatric office, hospital, or other clinical setting. However, using the population-based, public health approach widens the scope and role of mental health professionals. Rather than considering just the patient facing the clinician, the scope widens to that patient's family, social network, community, and neighborhood, and to society at large. Essentially, all of these entities become the patient, and interventions focus on improving mental health outcomes not only for the individual but for the families, communities, and societies within which the individual exists.

In addition to working within the health sector, public health emphasizes collaboration with other sectors that have an impact on health, including education, workplaces, the media, faith communities, government, and the justice system. The formation of interdisciplinary partnerships is key to improving mental health outcomes across populations.

Risk Factors and Protective Factors

Preventive interventions are based on determining and then addressing risk factors and protective factors, many of which are uncovered by social epidemiology. A risk factor is a characteristic that predates an adverse outcome (e.g., a mental illness) and is statistically associated with that outcome. Although it is not always the direct cause of the disorder, as a specific virus might be the cause of an infection, it is nevertheless associated with the disorder. A protective factor, likewise, is a characteristic that predates an adverse outcome and is associated with a reduced risk of developing that outcome. Thus, a risk factor increases the odds of a negative mental health outcome, whereas a protective factor decreases those odds. Some risk factors, such as low socioeconomic status or poor parenting skills, are malleable; others, such as age or family history, are not modifiable. Protective factors can also be malleable, as exemplified by the fact that a positive relationship between a child and a mentor or role model can increase that child's resiliency, serving as a buffer to current and future stressors (Rutter 1979).

Risk and protective factors can be proximal, meaning that they immediately precede or are closely timed in their association with mental health outcomes, or they can be distal and occur far "upstream" of the outcome. The social determinants of mental health can be seen as the distal risk factors, or the root causes, acting largely at the population level, which drive more proximal risk factors. In a groundbreaking article, Link and Phelan (1995) described these upstream risk factors as "the fundamental causes of disease," which they postulated would continue to exist even if more proximal risk factors and causes of disease were addressed. This conclusion highlights the broader social context involving social, cultural, political, and economic forces that increase risk, especially among vulnerable populations.

Evidence for such *fundamental* causes of disease has been clearly laid out by Marmot and Wilkinson (2006), who summarized the global evidence for the role of social factors in the development of disease and the persistence of health inequities. If risk factors such as unhealthy diet and unsafe living conditions are considered the precursors of disease, then the environmental and contextual factors that precede or shape these risk factors (e.g., food insecurity, inadequate enforcement of housing regulations) can be considered *the causes of the causes*. The fundamental causes, or the causes of the causes, are the social determinants of health and mental health, which can be mitigated through advocacy, political will, and policy interventions (Rose 1992; Marmot 2005). As we point out in this book, addressing social determinants is most effective through policy, although the more proximal social and environmental risk factors can also be considered at the programmatic and individual or clinical levels.

Mental Illness Prevention and Mental Health Promotion

Because the social determinants of mental health are considered fundamental, upstream, population-level causes, they are perhaps more relevant to prevention than to treatment. In the field of mental health, incorporating a preventive approach means considering risk and protective factors, the findings of public health and social epidemiology research, health promotion opportunities, evidence-based preventive interventions, and a population-based approach to the identification and management of mental illnesses. The increasing focus on prevention in mental health, and growth of the field of prevention science over the past 50 years, has been documented in Institute of Medicine reports. These publications describe long-term studies that have developed evidence-based programs to decrease risk factors and promote protective factors (Institute of Medicine 1994; Institute of Medicine and National Research Council 2009). Similar to mental illness prevention, mental health promotion is another concept in preventive psychiatry, defined as those interventions that increase health and well-being in populations (Commonwealth Department of Health and Aged Care 2000).

Gene-by-Environment Interactions and Epigenetics

Our deoxyribonucleic acid (DNA), variations in which play a prominent role in risk for many mental illnesses, does not exist in a vacuum. Accumulating research supports the views that genetic polymorphisms moderate the effects of socioenvironmental exposures (and vice versa) and that gene expression is affected by our environment and experiences (i.e., epigenetic effects) (Binder et al. 2008). As an example of the former, early adverse life experiences, chronic stress, abuse in its various forms, and neglect may interact with genetic susceptibilities, elevating risk for mental illnesses as varied as major depression and schizophrenia. Environment can also elevate risk through its effects on genetic structure and gene expression (National Scientific Council on the Developing Child 2005, 2010). Embracing the social determinants of mental health does not negate the importance of genetics in the causation of mental illnesses.

Intergenerational Perspective

The intergenerational perspective is imperative in understanding the social determinants of mental health. Social determinants are often transmitted from generation to generation, akin to autosomal dominant genetic transmission. Individuals born in poverty are significantly less likely to escape poverty in the current economic climate than in the past; reduced social mobility is an example of intergenerational transmission of social factors (Corcoran 1995). The intergenerational transmission of poor parenting, as well as adolescent problem behavior, teen pregnancy, and poverty, is well researched. These effects are mediated by parental factors (as well as other determinants), and addressing them may reduce and even prevent subsequent transmission (Conger et al. 1994; McLoyd 1998).

Mental Health Disparities, the Social Gradient, and the Pursuit of Social Justice

The social determinants of mental health are intimately linked to persistent inequities in the diagnosis, treatment, and management of mental illnesses. Physical health disparities have been thoroughly studied and defined over time (Smedley et al. 2009), but mental health disparities do not always follow the same patterns. Although rates of infant mortality, obesity, cardiovascular disease mortality, and early mortality are higher among minority populations compared with non-Hispanic whites (Mensah et al. 2005), rates of mental illnesses often are not significantly different across such groups. However, racial/ethnic minorities clearly have less access to and availability of mental health care and, when treated, tend to receive poorer-quality care. As a result, racial/ethnic minority populations experience a greater burden of disability associated with mental illnesses (U.S. Department of Health and Human Services 2001). In addition, socioeconomic status is as important in the conceptualization of disparities as race or ethnicity (Braveman et al. 2005; Kawachi et al. 2005; LaVeist and Wallace 2000). There is a general consensus that disparities in health and health care are driven largely by the social determinants of health. Disparities that exist in mental health are likewise driven by the social determinants of mental health.

Along these same lines, the concept of a *social gradient* indicates that the lower or worse one's position in society is, the worse one's health is likely to be. Those with higher positions in society are likely to enjoy better physical and mental health outcomes (Fisher and Baum 2010). Just as physical health has been robustly demonstrated to vary along a social gradient, mental health correlates strongly with one's position in society. The social gradient can be operationalized in numerous ways (e.g., on the basis of income, wealth, occupation, educational level, employment status, geographic location, or race/ethnicity). The social gradient in health relates prominently to differences in access to opportunity, power, and resources as well as varying exposure to stressors and social protective factors.

The term *social justice* is defined as the assurance that individuals in a society have equal opportunities to lead healthy, meaningful, productive, and empowered lives. Inequality in health is antithetical to social justice. We view the achieving of social justice as one of the great aspirations of society, and social justice can be considered the moral foundation of the field of public health (Powers and Faden 2008). As the Commission on Social Determinants of Health noted, "social injustice is killing people on a grand scale" (World Health Organization 2008, p. 26).

Limitations of the Social Determinants of the Mental Health Perspective

Despite the importance of the social determinants of mental health and a population-based, public health perspective, there are some caveats, limitations, and barriers to this approach to the prevention and treatment of mental illnesses; three will be briefly outlined here.

First, history tends to repeat itself, and the social determinants of mental health are not a novel concept. Previous decades have witnessed great enthusiasm (and perhaps excessive hope and optimism) in addressing the social determinants of mental health as a means of preventing mental illnesses. For example, the community mental health movement, which began roughly in the mid-1960s, viewed prevention as achievable by addressing social plights and injustices. However, despite these previous initiatives, limited progress has been made in addressing the social determinants of mental health. In this book, we aim to take an objective, balanced approach that is justifiably optimistic but not unduly buoyant.

Second, in exploring a topic as complex as the causes of mental illnesses in individuals and populations, it is all too easy to fall into an erroneous thought trap involving false dichotomies. The field of mental health has a storied history of generating and perpetuating deceivingly polar explanations (e.g., the nature vs. nurture debate noted above). For instance, to provide a rough sketch of the intellectual history behind the etiology of schizophrenia, following Kraepelin, there was a frantic search for the biological *cause* of schizophrenia. When this came up short (at least partially because of the lack of appropriate neurobiological methods at the time), the field swung to the assumption that etiology must be *social* and thus attributable to the family dynamic (e.g., the schizophrenogenic mother). Only recently have psychiatrists been able to recognize that the onset and course of mental illnesses are caused and influenced by a complex interaction of congenital, biological, environmental, and social factors. When discussing the social determinants of mental health, there is a risk of similar false dichotomies. For instance, when thinking about poverty, it is tempting for some people to assume that the poor are either entirely helpless victims of their circumstances or are to blame for their own poverty because of poor choices influenced by a culture of poverty. In fact, as chapters in this book will elucidate, poverty indeed victimizes people in ways that limit their choices, damage their communities, and harm their mental health, at times perpetuating poverty itself (which can seem like a culture of poverty when viewed out of context). Thus, a balanced approach is required when considering the social determinants of mental health.

Third, the social determinants of mental health concept might be seen as placing the blame of causing poor mental health on society at large; however, we do not discount the important role of personal choice and health behaviors. With increasing epidemiological data, the public has become more aware of the impact of lifestyle choices on health outcomes. Examples of this include the impact of cigarette smoking, unhealthy diet, and sedentary lifestyle on cardiovascular disease, cancer, diabetes, and chronic obstructive pulmonary disease. Although all of these conditions have complex genetic underpinnings and measurable biological correlates, the role of the social environment in the development and course of these diseases is indisputable. For example, we know that the risk of developing diabetes is strongly influenced by calorie-dense, high-sugar, high-fat, and micronutrient-poor diets. But what causes individuals to choose diets replete with sugar, fat, and salt? And to what extent is it really an active choice? Social, economic, and environmental factors strongly shape and constrict food choices. Individuals who are poor may choose more inexpensive, energy-dense foods because that is what is available to them. Low-income neighborhoods may have limited food options or may be overrun by fast food restaurants that advertise extensively in those communities, especially to children (Andreyeva et al. 2011). Furthermore, chronic stress associated with adverse life experiences is associated with consumption of an unhealthy diet. What initially appears to be individual choice is, on further analysis, embedded in the complex social and physical context in which people make their choices and live their lives. In certain contexts, choice is severely restricted, and barriers to making healthy choices are unfairly high.

Earlier Informative Theoretical Frameworks

To appropriately conceptualize the social determinants of mental health and to prevent a gap between rhetoric and reality in terms of implementing approaches to address the social determinants, a clear but comprehensive theoretical framework is needed (Larsson 2013). Because concepts pertaining to the social determinants of mental health have existed for many years, previous theoretical models have guided our own.

The social ecological model, originally conceptualized by Bronfenbrenner, describes a multilevel, dynamic interrelationship between individuals and the social environment. Specifically, Bronfenbrenner's ecological framework comprises the individual, microsystem, mesosystem, exosystem, and macrosystem and how an individual interacts with these systemic layers within society (Bronfenbrenner 1977). Over time, multiple revisions to the social ecological model have resulted in changing terminologies, with system levels being reframed in various ways (e.g., relationship, neighborhood, community, and society levels). Similarly, Dahlgren and Whitehead (1993) created a widely cited conceptual framework that depicts the determinants of health in what they described as layers of influence on an individual's health potential. These layers include individual lifestyle factors; social and community networks; living and working conditions; and general socioeconomic, cultural, and environmental conditions. As in the social ecological model, the individual is the center of the framework, and the policy-relevant influences surround the individual. These models effectively depict the various layers of the social environment around the individual and have increased understanding of the importance of the social determinants of health.

Healthy People 2020 (a U.S. federal document that provides science-based, 10-year national objectives for improving the health of all Americans) elevated the social determinants of health to a topic area of interest and developed a *place-based* comprehensive framework to describe the social determinants of health (Office of Disease Prevention and Health Promotion 2014). The five key determinants identified by *Healthy People 2020* are economic stability, education, social and community context, health and health care, and neighborhood and built environment. Within each of these areas, key issues were identified. For example, in considering economic stability in depth, poverty, employment status, access to employment, and housing stability were identified. For the neighborhood and built environment, quality of housing, crime and violence, environmental conditions, and access to healthy foods were described. This framework helps organize a very large topic area into more digestible, basic components, but it does not highlight the complex interconnections between them.

The Commission on Social Determinants of Health was established by the World Health Organization in 2005 to advance health equity and address the gaping, persistent inequalities in health worldwide. As part of its charge, the commission developed a comprehensive, action-oriented framework to facilitate addressing the social determinants of health. The commission described structural determinants (socioeconomic position, governance structures, public policies, and sociocultural values and norms) and intermediary determinants (material living and working conditions, behaviors and biology, and psychosocial factors) and emphasized the bidirectional relationships between these two major domains of determinants. This framework highlights the relevance of various policies, including those that are not typically considered "health policies" per se, to health outcomes of populations (Todman and Diaz 2014). However, the exclusion of mental health in the discourse and development of this framework is a limitation for our purposes.

Framework for Conceptualizing the Social Determinants of Mental Health

In building on the various frameworks that provide a theoretical grounding for our understanding of the social determinants, we present a model that considers the social determinants of mental health from a multilevel perspective. It benefits from, and is intended to build on, the aforementioned frameworks. Figure 1–1 shows the driving forces behind social, environmental, and behavioral risk factors for poor physical and mental health as well as disease and morbidity. In reviewing this architecture of risk, we will begin by describing the deepest layers.

Society Unwell: Public Policies and Social Norms Underlie the Social Determinants

At the most foundational level, the factors that drive ultimate health risk can be characterized by two types of ubiquitous, pervasive, and persistent (and perhaps even difficult to recognize as pertinent to health) social contextual factors: *public policies* and *social norms.* The former factor includes policies, codes, rules, and legislation pertaining to education, employment, wages, food, housing, neighborhoods, and many other facets of society. Examples include the tuition costs for higher education within a state's college system, federal minimum wage legislation, and city and county zoning ordinances. These public policies usually do not appear to be health policies, but as we will see across the chapters in this book, they drive the social determinants of mental health, which in turn drive risk and, ultimately, mental health outcomes.

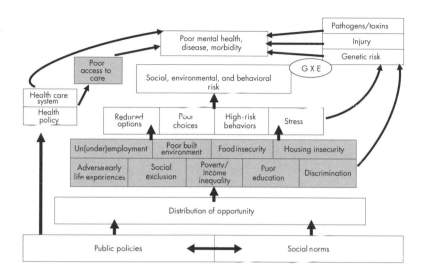

FIGURE 1-1. Framework for understanding the social determinants of mental health.

G × E = gene-by-environment interaction.

Whereas public policies are codified, social norms pertain to values, attitudes, impressions, and biases. As such, social norms are largely learned and promulgated within groups, are not officiated, and can exert their effects unconsciously. Rather than regulations, they are opinions and beliefs, including political ideologies as well as views on class, race or ethnicity, and gender, to name just a few. These norms typically would not be thought of as determinants of health and disease, but they—along with their public policy counterparts—are driving forces behind many of the social determinants of mental health and thus underlie risk factors and, ultimately, health outcomes.

We believe that the greatest population-based impact on health and disease would be achieved by acting at this level, that is, by optimizing public policies to make them more health promoting and by altering social norms so that together we prioritize the health of all members of society. To heal an unwell society, we must carefully evaluate our public policies and begin to shift social norms.

Society Unfair: Unequal Distribution of Opportunity Drives the Social Determinants

Both public policies and social norms tend to favor some individuals and some groups over others, which sets the stage for an unequal distribution of opportunities. Inequalities, exemplified by income inequality (Wilkinson and Pickett 2009), are known to underpin many, if not most, health conditions. Inequality is driven by regulations (public policies) and opinions (social norms), and inequality is a driving force behind most of the core social determinants of health. Although income inequality is perhaps the best-studied form of inequality, the unequal distribution of opportunity is also apparent in terms of education, political voice, and other aspects of civic life.

Many of the social determinants of health that will receive individual attention in subsequent chapters of this book come about largely through inequalities. For example, food insecurity in the United States is grounded not in a shortage of food but in an unequal distribution of and access to adequate, healthy food (Carlson et al. 1999). Food insecurity and the other issues addressed in these chapters, which might be considered the core social determinants of mental health (depicted in Figure 1–1 as unemployment or underemployment, poor education, discrimination and social exclusion, neighborhood disorder, adverse early life experiences, food insecurity, and housing instability), can have both direct and indirect effects on health outcomes (although, in order to reduce unnecessary complexity, these are not shown separately in the figure). That is, in addition to direct effects on health (e.g., adverse early life experiences causing physical injury, food insecurity leading to micronutrient deficiencies, poor housing quality causing exposure to lead or other neurotoxins, neighborhood disorder leading to gun violence–related injuries), these core social determinants have diverse indirect effects on health as well.

Although the direct effects on health might seem straightforward and easy to identify, the core social determinants of mental health have more pernicious effects on health through their indirect effects. Specifically, they lead to stress (which is associated with cascading psychological and physiological pathways to disease), they lead to poor choices and risky behaviors (e.g., problematic alcohol use, overeating, and not engaging in physical activity), and, importantly, they constrict choice among those affected (e.g., low income and food insecurity are associated with reliance on an inexpensive, calorie-dense, and unhealthy diet). We conceptualize the social determinants of poor mental health and elevated risk for mental illnesses as a risk architecture with a foundation of problematic public policies and social norms that lead to unfair distribution of opportunity.

We have emphasized the often covert role of public policies; however, actual health policies are obviously also important to consider. Health policies shape the structure and function of the health care system, which clearly has an impact on individual and population health and disease. Poor access to health care (which we conceptualize as another of the core social determinants of mental health) therefore has an important role in shaping health and disease.

Although Figure 1–1 focuses primarily on the driving social forces behind social, environmental, and behavioral risk factors (which in turn directly contribute to disease), we readily acknowledge the importance of genetic risk—and gene-by-environment interactions—as well. Furthermore, in addition to socioenvironmental and genetic risk, both physical and mental health are affected by certain events and exposures, such as injury and pathogens or toxins. Although at first glance those causative agents might seem irrelevant to a discussion of social determinants of health, the individual's and the community's likelihood of such exposures is, in fact, unequally distributed, and that unfair distribution is intimately linked to the social determinants of health.

Our framework suggests that risk for poor mental health and mental illnesses can be most broadly and effectively minimized by working at the deepest levels. As we conceptualize nongenetic (socioenvironmental) causation, poor choices and risky behaviors are closely tied to stress and constricted choice, which are driven first by diverse social determinants of mental health. These social determinants are in turn driven by unequal distribution of opportunity (inequality), which is driven ultimately by public policies and social norms. Although we must intervene at all levels, the deeper we go, the greater the overall impact will be.

Call to Action

Even though we often deal with the end result of many risk factors when providing direct patient care, we must also consider upstream factors, the causes of the causes, and the socioenvironmental context, which ultimately lead to each patient's presentation in the clinical setting. In a health care environment that is increasingly pressed for time, in which psychiatrists' roles are often reduced to rapid medication checks, we need to move from a culture of witnessing the negative impact of the social environment on mental health and thinking "someone should do something about this" to "I should do something about this" and, finally, "I can do something about this." Through community involvement to shift social norms and through engagement with the legislative process to improve public policy, we can experience a sense of community-focused agency, promote a more equal distribution of opportunity, and begin to heal an unfair and unwell society.

Key Points

- The social determinants of mental health are those conditions in which we are born, grow, live, work, and age that have an impact on our mental health and are shaped by the distribution of money, power, and resources in society.

- The social determinants of mental health are largely responsible for inequalities in the toll that mental illnesses take on subsets of the population. For this reason, attention to the social determinants of mental health is a moral imperative.

- Central to the social determinants of mental health approach is shifting the concept of mental illnesses from an individual patient approach to a public health, population-based approach.

- At the most foundational level, the factors that drive the social determinants of mental health are public policies and social norms, which set the stage for the unequal distribution of opportunity.

- Psychiatrists and other mental health professionals have a responsibility to identify and address the causes of the causes of mental illnesses, the social determinants of mental health.

References

Andreyeva T, Kelly IR, Harris JL: Exposure to food advertising on television: associations with children's fast food and soft drink consumption and obesity. Econ Hum Biol 9(3):221–233, 2011 21439918

Binder EB, Bradley RG, Liu W, et al: Association of FKBP5 polymorphisms and childhood abuse with risk of posttraumatic stress disorder symptoms in adults. JAMA 299(11):1291–1305, 2008 18349090

Braveman PA, Cubbin C, Egerter S, et al: Socioeconomic status in health research: one size does not fit all. JAMA 294(22):2879–2888, 2005 16352796

Breslau N, Kessler RC, Chilcoat HD, et al: Trauma and posttraumatic stress disorder in the community: the 1996 Detroit Area Survey of Trauma. Arch Gen Psychiatry 55(7):626–632, 1998 9672053

Bronfenbrenner U: Toward an experimental ecology of human development. Am Psychol 32:513–531, 1977

Carlson SJ, Andrews MS, Bickel GW: Measuring food insecurity and hunger in the United States: development of a national benchmark measure and prevalence estimates. J Nutr 129(2S)(suppl):510S–516S, 1999 10064320

Centers for Disease Control and Prevention: Social Determinants of Health. Atlanta, GA, Centers for Disease Control and Prevention, 2014. Available at: http://www.cdc.gov/socialdeterminants. Accessed June 20, 2014.

Commonwealth Department of Health and Aged Care: National Action Plan for Promotion, Prevention and Early Intervention for Mental Health. Canberra, Commonwealth Department of Health and Aged Care, 2000

Conger RD, Ge X, Elder GH Jr, et al: Economic stress, coercive family process, and developmental problems of adolescents. Child Dev 65(2 Spec No):541–561, 1994 8013239

Corcoran M: Rags to rags: Poverty and mobility in the United States. Annu Rev Sociol 21:237–267, 1995

Dahlgren G, Whitehead M: Tackling inequalities in health: what can we learn from what has been tried? Working paper prepared for the King's Fund International Seminar on Tackling Inequalities in Health. London, King's Fund, 1993

Donley S, Habib L, Jovanovic T, et al: Civilian PTSD symptoms and risk for involvement in the criminal justice system. J Am Acad Psychiatry Law 40(4):522–529, 2012 23233474

Durkheim E: Suicide: A Study in Sociology (1897). Translated by Spaulding JA, Simpson G. Glencoe, IL, Free Press, 1951

Ferrari AJ, Charlson FJ, Norman RE, et al: Burden of depressive disorders by country, sex, age, and year: findings from the global burden of disease study 2010. PLoS Med 10(11):e1001547, 2013 24223526

Fisher M, Baum F: The social determinants of mental health: implications for research and health promotion. Aust N Z J Psychiatry 44(12):1057–1063, 2010 20973623

Goodell S, Druss B, Walker ER: Mental Disorders and Medical Comorbidity. Princeton, NJ, Robert Wood Johnson Foundation, 2011

Insel TR, Landis SC, Collins FS: The NIH BRAIN Initiative: research priorities. Science 340(6133):687–688, 2013 23661744

Institute of Medicine: Reducing Risks for Mental Disorders: Frontiers for Preventive Intervention Research. Washington, DC, National Academy Press, 1994

Institute of Medicine and National Research Council: Preventing Mental, Emotional, and Behavioral Disorders Among Young People: Progress and Possibilities. Washington, DC, National Academies Press, 2009

Jakupcak M, Cook J, Imel Z, et al: Posttraumatic stress disorder as a risk factor for suicidal ideation in Iraq and Afghanistan War veterans. J Trauma Stress 22(4):303–306, 2009 19626682

Kawachi I, Daniels N, Robinson DE: Health disparities by race and class: why both matter. Health Aff (Millwood) 24(2):343–352, 2005 15757918

Kessler RC, Berglund P, Demler O, et al: Lifetime prevalence and age-of-onset distributions of DSM-IV disorders in the National Comorbidity Survey Replication. Arch Gen Psychiatry 62(6):593–602, 2005 15939837

Larsson P: The rhetoric/reality gap in social determinants of mental health. Mental Health Review Journal 18:182–193, 2013

LaVeist TA, Wallace JM Jr: Health risk and inequitable distribution of liquor stores in African American neighborhood. Soc Sci Med 51(4):613–617, 2000 10868674

Link BG, Phelan J: Social conditions as fundamental causes of disease. J Health Soc Behav 35(Spec No):80–94, 1995 7560851

Marmot M: Social determinants of health inequalities. Lancet 365(9464):1099–1104, 2005 15781105

Marmot M, Wilkinson RG: Social Determinants of Health, 2nd Edition. Oxford, UK, Oxford University Press, 2006

McLoyd VC: Socioeconomic disadvantage and child development. Am Psychol 53(2):185–204, 1998 9491747

Mensah GA, Mokdad AH, Ford ES, et al: State of disparities in cardiovascular health in the United States. Circulation 111(10):1233–1241, 2005 15769763

National Scientific Council on the Developing Child: Excessive Stress Disrupts the Architecture of the Developing Brain, Working Paper No 3. Cambridge, MA, Center on the Developing Child, 2005

National Scientific Council on the Developing Child: Early Experiences Can Alter Gene Expression and Affect Long-Term Development, Working Paper No 10. Cambridge, MA, Center on the Developing Child, 2010

Office of Disease Prevention and Health Promotion: Social Determinants. Washington, D.C., U.S. Department of Health and Human Services, 2014. Available at: http://www.healthypeople.gov/2020/leading-health-indicators/2020-lhi-topics/social-determinants. Accessed October 10, 2014.

Parks J, Svendsen D, Singer P, et al (eds): Morbidity and Mortality in People With Serious Mental Illness. Alexandria, VA, National Association of State Mental Health Program Directors Medical Directors Council, 2006

Powers M, Faden R: Social Justice: The Moral Foundations of Public Health and Health Policy. New York, Oxford University Press, 2008

Reese C, Pederson T, Avila S, et al: Screening for traumatic stress among survivors of urban trauma. J Trauma Acute Care Surg 73(2):462–467, discussion 467–468, 2012 22846957

Rose G: The Strategy of Preventive Medicine. Oxford, UK, Oxford University Press, 1992

Rutter M: Protective factors in children's responses to stress and disadvantage. Ann Acad Med Singapore 8(3):324–338, 1979 547874

Smedley BD, Stith AY, Nelson AR: Unequal Treatment: Confronting Racial and Ethnic Disparities in Health Care. Washington, DC, National Academies Press, 2009

Todman LC, Diaz A: A public health approach to narrowing mental health disparities. Psychiatr Ann 44:27–31, 2014

Torrey EF: Jails and prisons—America's new mental hospitals. Am J Public Health 85(12):1611–1613, 1995 7503330

U.S. Department of Health and Human Services: Mental Health: A Report of the Surgeon General. Rockville, MD, Substance Abuse and Mental Health Services Administration, 1999

U.S. Department of Health and Human Services: Mental Health: Culture, Race, and Ethnicity—A Supplement to Mental Health: A Report of the Surgeon General. Rockville, MD, Substance Abuse and Mental Health Services Administration, 2001

Wilkinson R, Pickett K: Income inequality and social dysfunction. Annu Rev Sociol 35:493–511, 2009

World Health Organization: Closing the Gap in a Generation: Health Equity Through Action on the Social Determinants of Health. Geneva, Switzerland, Commission on Social Determinants of Health, 2008

World Health Organization: Addressing the Social Determinants of Health: The Urban Dimension and the Role of Local Government. Edited by Grady M, Goldblatt P. Copenhagen, Regional Office for Europe, 2012

Wu S, Green A: Projection of Chronic Illness Prevalence and Cost Inflation. Santa Monica, CA, RAND Health, 2000

2

Discrimination

Jane A. Rafferty, M.A.
Jamie M. Abelson, M.S.W.
Kimson Bryant, B.A.
James S. Jackson, Ph.D.

No one is born hating another person because of the color of his skin, or his background, or his religion. People must learn to hate, and if they can learn to hate, they can be taught to love, for love comes more naturally to the human heart than its opposite.

Nelson Mandela, 1918–2013

There is growing interest in, and recognition of, the association between discrimination and health problems (Williams et al. 2003). Some research suggests a positive change in racial attitudes in the United States, with whites reporting increasing support for racial equality (Schuman et al. 1997), and there are recent narratives about a postracial society. How-

The authors express sincere appreciation to Julie Sweetman for her assistance with the analyses and sourcing and acknowledge the greater support of the Program for Research on Black Americans. Support was provided in part by the MacArthur and Robert Wood Johnson Foundations and the National Institute on Minority Health and Health Disparities (NIMHD).

ever, a range of evidence points to the persistence of the salience of race in people's attitudes and behaviors, as well as continuing institutional forms of racism and discrimination. Survey data show that although there is increasing support for the principle of racial equality, there is less endorsement of actual programs intended to ameliorate racial inequality (Bobo and Kluegel 1993). Furthermore, institutional racism persists; for example, audit studies suggest that similarly qualified black and white job applicants are not treated equally, with whites being more likely to get an interview or to be hired (Pager and Shepherd 2008). Although discrimination within the housing market has been illegal since the Fair Housing Act of 1968, residential segregation persists; that is, most neighborhoods are characterized by a high concentration of one racial/ethnic group or another (Glaeser and Vigdor 2012; Massey and Denton 1993). Finally, the extent of racial inequalities in arrests and convictions translates into disproportionate representation of ethnic and racial minority groups in the criminal justice system (Alexander 2010).

In light of the evidence suggesting the persistence of the salience of race in American society, the study of discrimination represents a compelling theoretical and empirical lens with which to consider disparities in health and risk for both physical and mental illnesses. Discrimination in its multiple forms (e.g., discrimination based on color or race, age, gender, or sexual orientation) is an important social determinant of health and may be linked to other social determinants, including gender and socioeconomic status, perhaps forming fundamental causes of poor health (Link and Phelan 1995; Phelan et al. 2010).

This chapter includes three sections. First, we begin with an overview of discrimination and effective ways to measure discrimination, especially in social surveys. We place the study of discrimination in the larger context of the long-standing, interlocking streams of research undertaken to understand social gradients in health by linking social and demographic contexts to the concept of stress and, in turn, to health outcomes (Jackson et al. 2003). In our research, we have used the 2001–2003 National Survey of American Life (NSAL) to empirically examine some basic associations between measures of chronic stress and discrimination and the prevalence of specific mental disorders. Second, we turn to the clinical setting and outline broad strategies behavioral health clinicians can employ to assess a patient's social and cultural context and to explore a patient's exposure to various forms of stress, including discrimination. Third, we review a range of policy recommendations, essentially concluding that although ample policies and guidelines have been established, especially since 1964, widespread, effective enforcement remains an elusive goal.

Although prejudice, discrimination, and social exclusion of any sort are likely damaging to both physical and mental health, we will focus specifically on race-based discrimination to make our points. We assume that the psychological and physiological stress mechanisms underpinning other forms of discrimination (e.g., discrimination based on sexual orientation) are the same as or similar to those associated with race-based discrimination. Additionally, in this chapter we focus more specifically on the impact of discrimination on black populations including individuals of African and of Caribbean descent; we recognize that there are unique issues related to discrimination that many racial and ethnic groups face in the United States and that these experiences vary in complex ways. Our examination of racial discrimination (and focus on African Americans and black Caribbeans) is warranted given the long history and ongoing state of racial inequality in the United States and the fact that racial inequality has been studied more than other forms of discrimination and social exclusion.

Discrimination and Mental Health: An Overview

Racial Group Discrimination in the United States

We define race primarily as a socially constructed characteristic based on physical attributes and ancestry (Cogburn et al. 2013; Griffin and Jackson 2009). Racism represents a set of social arrangements that translates the classification of individuals into a social hierarchy of privilege and opportunity. Two social consequences of racism are the development of negative attitudes or prejudices and differential treatment by racial group, or discrimination. The latter can exist at both individual and institutional levels (Bonilla-Silva 1997; Clark et al. 1999; Krieger 2012; Williams and Mohammed 2009; Williams et al. 1997) and can be both consciously intended and unintentional (Tyrer 2005).

Although some dimensions of race transcend national context, it is instructive to consider national and historical variation in the United States. Comparative analyses point to differences in the meaning of race. In the United States, one is classified as black if one has any known black ancestry. In contrast, for example, the Brazilian system of racial classification is more fluid, depending on phenotypic characteristics of individuals (Omi and Winant 1994; Telles 2004). Key historical legacies in the United States include legalized forms of a racial caste, including slavery and the subsequent Jim Crow laws established in the last quarter of the nineteenth century and lasting until the mid-twentieth century. The mid- to late twentieth century witnessed notable landmark court rulings and essential legislation that represented important civil rights victories, including *Brown v. Board of Education* in 1954, the Civil Rights Act of 1964, and the Voting Rights Act of 1965. However, many social markers, including unequal educational attainment and income, residential segregation, disparities in physical and mental health, and overrepresentation of black Americans, Hispanics, and Latinos in the criminal justice system, collectively indicate that deep divisions among racial and ethnic groups persist and that enforcement of existing legislation is far from complete (Alexander 2010; Fischer and Hout 2006).

We position our evaluation of the impact of discrimination on health within existing streams of research across many fields of social science, public health, and natural science. Common across this work is an implicit framework that seeks to understand the links among social conditions, the concept of stress, and health status. This framework is in sharp contrast to the mid-twentieth-century perspective that viewed incidence and prevalence of disease as a function of solely biological processes and medical care (House 2002). Hans Selye was a pioneer in the study of stress; he identified a set of processes linking noxious social, psychological, or physical stimuli to physiological responses originating in the hypothalamic-pituitary-adrenal axis and sympathetic nervous system (Selye 1956). In the presence of a stressor, the body shifts into fight-or-flight mode, and the hypothalamic-pituitary-adrenal axis is activated, resulting in elevated cortisol, as well as increased heart rate and blood pressure. Selye postulated that following prolonged exposure, certain stimuli could lead to the onset of diseases such as cardiovascular disease.

This biological framework led to the development of concepts of stress that varied from discrete (i.e., acute traumatic events) to continuous (i.e., chronic sources of stress). Examples of acute events include experiencing the death of a loved one or being physically assaulted. In contrast, examples of chronic or day-to-day stress include problems or worries within one's family or the presence of financial problems (House 2002; Lazarus and Folkman 1984; Pearlin 1989).

There is a broad range of conceptualizations of discrimination (Brown 2001; Kressin et al. 2008; Landrine and Klonoff 1996). In our work, we measure discrimination by assessing experiences of unfair treatment across a range of life domains. Following the conceptual distinction in previous work on stress, we identify acute (or major) kinds of discrimination and chronic (or everyday) forms of discrimination.

Acute, major experiences of discrimination describe those in a variety of domains of life such as being unfairly fired or being unfairly prevented from moving into a neighborhood. Everyday, chronic discrimination captures a range of day-to-day experiences such as being followed around in stores or being treated with less respect than others. Categories of attribution or the reason for the discrimination include race, age, sex, and weight. A common metric for measuring discrimination is a count of the number of life domains in which an individual has experienced discrimination (Williams et al. 2012a, 2012b).

Discrimination as a Social Determinant of Health

A growing body of work examines the effects of discrimination on physical health. Commonly studied health outcomes include blood pressure and cardiovascular disease, self-reported measures of health conditions, overall self-rated health, and mortality rates. Although findings are largely consistent in some areas, in others, the various examinations of associations have produced mixed results.

Results on the relationship between discrimination and blood pressure are somewhat mixed. In laboratory-based research, participants were exposed to situations or stimuli conveying racist events, and then their blood pressure reactivity was assessed. The results suggested that exposure to racist events results in elevated blood pressure (Clark 2006; Richman et al. 2007; Williams and Mohammed 2009). However, in community studies assessing experiences with discrimination and high blood pressure, the results were mixed; thus, it appears that the relationship between discrimination and sustained high blood pressure is complex. In some studies, researchers found no association (Williams and Mohammed 2009), and in one study, a nonlinear relationship between reports of discrimination and systolic blood pressure was found (Ryan et al. 2006). Ryan and colleagues showed that respondents reporting some experience with discrimination had lower systolic blood pressure than those reporting no experience with discrimination, but respondents reporting high levels of discrimination had the highest levels of blood pressure.

Research on the effect of discrimination on cardiovascular disease is also equivocal. In a multicity study of menopausal women, Lewis and colleagues (2006) found a relationship between chronic or everyday discrimination and the presence of coronary artery calcification. Results from a national study that examined the relationship between experiences of acute or major discrimination and self-reports of cardiovascular disease among African American men did not reveal a statistically significant association between discrimination and a diagnosis of cardiovascular disease (defined as at least one of the following: hypertension, atherosclerosis, myocardial infarction, or stroke) (Chae et al. 2010). However, agreement with negative racial stereotypes regarding African Americans (e.g., they are lazy, they are likely to give up easily, they are violent), moderated the effect of discrimination on cardiovascular health. Among African American men who scored low on negative racial group attitudes, there was a nonlinear relationship between discrimination and reports of cardiovascular disease. Specifically, the probability of a history of cardiovascular disease was highest among respondents reporting two situations of discrimination, and the probability was lower among those with fewer reports of discrimination, as well as among those reporting three or more reports of discrimination. However, among African American men who scored high on negative racial group attitudes, the same relationship is also nonlinear, but with a different pattern: respondents reporting two experiences of discrimination had the lowest probability of having had cardiovascular disease. These results parallel findings of Krieger and Sidney (1996) among working-class African American men. Overall, these works suggest that beliefs regarding one's racial group have the potential either to buffer or to exacerbate the effects of the experience of discrimination on the risk for cardiovascular disease; the health risks of discrimination vary depending on one's own level of internalized racism.

A range of studies assessing other health outcomes suggests fairly consistent associations with discrimination, including assessments of self-reported health (Williams et al. 1997), reported chronic conditions (Gee et al. 2007), and mortality rates (Barnes et al. 2008; Williams et al. 2003). Across these studies, discrimination was found to be predictive of poorer health status.

Discrimination as a Social Determinant of Mental Health

Discrimination is also associated with poorer mental health outcomes. Using the NSAL, a unique national data set that allows for consideration of racial and ethnic group differences, we empirically explored some of the associations between discrimination and mental health that have been identified in earlier studies (Williams et al. 2003). We ran analyses separately for four race/ethnicity/nativity groups (African Americans, U.S.-born black Caribbeans, foreign-born black Caribbeans, and non-Hispanic whites), controlling for a range of individual-level demographic and socioeconomic indicators (age, sex, region of residence, marital status, education, and poverty status).

The summary of lifetime mood measure captures whether one meets criteria in one's lifetime for at least one of four depressive and mood disorders (major depressive disorder, persistent depressive disorder [dysthymia], bipolar I disorder, or bipolar II disorder).[1] Similarly, the summary lifetime anxiety measure represents whether one has met criteria in one's lifetime for one of four anxiety disorders (panic disorder, agoraphobia without panic disorder, social anxiety disorder [social phobia], or generalized anxiety disorder). The chronic stress measure represents the number of domains of day-to-day life that represent sources of stress (e.g., health, employment, family life).We assessed experiences of discrimination in 9 acute (or major) life areas and in 10 chronic (or everyday) life domains (see Tables 2–1 and 2–2); for each we examined race-based and non-race-based measures of discrimination.

In predicting lifetime depressive and mood disorders and lifetime anxiety disorders across all race/ethnicity/nativity groups, chronic stress is a consistent predictor; that is, reporting stress in more domains of life is associated with a greater likelihood of meeting criteria for at least one lifetime depressive or mood disorder and also for at least one lifetime anxiety disorder. Overall, experience with race-based major discrimination is a more consistent predictor of lifetime depressive and mood disorders than lifetime anxiety disorders. Reporting at least one experience of major race-based discrimination is associated with higher odds of meeting criteria for a lifetime depressive or mood disorder. The effects of everyday discrimination are a bit more limited, although we do find some statistically significant effects. Among African Americans and in both black Caribbean groups, having at least one everyday discrimination experience attributed to race is associated with a greater likelihood of meeting criteria for at least one lifetime anxiety disorder. Among African Americans and foreign-born black Caribbeans, there is a positive association with race-based everyday discrimination and meeting criteria for a lifetime depressive or mood disorder. Overall, analyses show that among blacks, experiencing discriminatory circumstances is associated with higher odds of reporting depressive, mood, and anxiety disorders.

---

[1]The disorder measures used in these analyses were based on DSM-IV criteria.

TABLE 2–1. National Survey of American Life major discrimination domains

At any time in your life, have you ever been *unfairly* fired?

For *unfair* reasons, have you ever not been hired for a job?

Have you ever been *unfairly* denied a promotion?

Have you ever been *unfairly* prevented from moving into a neighborhood because the landlord or a realtor refused to sell or rent you a house or apartment?

Have you ever moved into a neighborhood where neighbors made life difficult for you or your family?

Have you ever been *unfairly* denied a bank loan?

Have you ever received service from someone such as a plumber or car mechanic that was worse than what other people get?

Have you ever been *unfairly* discouraged by a teacher or advisor from continuing your education?

Have you ever been *unfairly* stopped, searched, questioned, physically threatened, or abused by the police?

Source. Jackson et al. 2001–2003

TABLE 2–2. National Survey of American Life everyday discrimination domains

You are treated with less courtesy than other people.

You are treated with less respect than other people.

You receive poorer service than other people at restaurants or stores.

People act as if they think you are not smart.

People act as if they are afraid of you.

People act as if they think you are dishonest.

People act as if they are better than you are.

You are called names or insulted.

You are threatened or harassed.

You are followed around in stores.

Source. Jackson et al. 2001–2003

In addition to the analyses that we have done with the NSAL, several studies also highlight the association between stress, discrimination, and poor mental health (Brown et al. 2000; Karlsen and Nazroo 2002; LaVeist 1996; Levine et al. 2014; Pascoe and Smart Richman 2009). For example, race-based job discrimination can have mental health effects, such as elevated levels of psychological distress and a lowered sense of mastery and control (Krieger 1990). Work by Soto et al. (2011) demonstrated that all forms of discrimination are associated with generalized anxiety disorder, but, predictably, race-based discrimination is five times more prevalent for blacks than whites and is thus a significant predictor of this anxiety disorder among African Americans.

Chronic Stress and Racial Group Discrimination: Approaches for the Clinical Setting

Case Example: Damaging Effects of Chronic Stress and Discrimination

Kevin Franklin is a 28-year-old, single African American male reluctantly seeking evaluation and treatment from a local university psychiatry clinic. Dr. Brianna Bates, a third-year psychiatry resident, performs an initial evaluation. Mr. Franklin claims, "My girlfriend said she'd leave me if I didn't talk to someone." Mr. Franklin acknowledges that he has had a tough life but insists that his upbringing was not extraordinary and he is fine now. Dr. Bates asks about his girlfriend's complaints. Mr. Franklin says that she thinks that he is avoiding her, that he is not looking for a job, and that he is spending too much time on the computer and drinking with his buddies.

Until a few years ago, Mr. Franklin had been working on the assembly line at a vehicle manufacturing plant, but he was laid off during the recession. After searching for several months, he was unable to find another job, and he eventually started spending more time at home watching television and hanging out with old friends. He acknowledges to Dr. Bates that they do a lot of drinking, but he thinks he can handle it. Pressed for details, he admits that he actually has not been spending as much time with his friends anymore and is now spending more time drinking alone. When Dr. Bates seeks more information, Mr. Franklin notes that he has little energy, that he sleeps more than usual, and that he and his friends have been hanging out in places that have brought back some bad memories. Mr. Franklin acknowledges that the neighborhood he grew up in was "pretty rough," he "lost some good friends," and the memories still make him "kind of jumpy." Therefore, he feels that he is better off just hanging out alone, drinking a beer and watching a movie. He liked staying at his girlfriend's house, but he says that it is now less satisfying because she keeps asking him about applying for jobs, telling him that he is depressed, and encouraging him to get help. Mr. Franklin admits that he is getting tired of his girlfriend's "constant pestering." He tells Dr. Bates that he came in to placate his girlfriend, even though he believes that no psychiatrist can help him find a job.

Mr. Franklin acknowledges to Dr. Bates that his mood is low and he has no hope that things will get better any time soon. He also sleeps excessively during the daytime and is often awake at night. When asked about the old neighborhood, his memories, and feeling jumpy, he tells Dr. Bates that "bad things happen on the streets" and that he has learned to always be vigilant. When Dr. Bates specifically questions him, he reveals that he often reacts intensely to unexpected sounds, erupts emotionally to even mild frustrations, and yells more than he wants to when interacting with his girlfriend. Recently, he had been angry about an experience of "driving while black." He recounts that a police officer pulled him over for no discernible reason when he was on his way to pick up his girlfriend after a graduate class she was attending. He was late to meet her, she complained, and they had a verbal altercation; now he regrets having taken out his frustration on her.

After hearing about this recent incident with the police, Dr. Bates asks Mr. Franklin about other experiences of discrimination. He recalls that as teens, he and his friends were regularly hassled by the police. Throughout high school, he observed that his white friends never invited him over to their houses or accepted an invitation to his, even though he knew they were spending time at each other's houses outside of school. And when he had been working and making good money, he felt he was sometimes treated badly by store clerks who did not seem to believe he had money to spend and often followed him around the store while he shopped. He also says that he wonders if his being laid off was tied to his being black; however, he recognizes that many people lost their jobs at that time. More recently, he has been wondering if discrimination is part of the reason why he has not been able to get a new job. He applied for some jobs for which he knew he was qualified but was rarely invited for an interview. Additionally, more than once, he was called in for an interview and then was told when he arrived that the position had already been filled.

Mr. Franklin tells Dr. Bates that he grew up in poverty, pretty much raising himself. His parents used drugs. He made money dealing drugs for a while but stopped doing so when his brother died. (He did not want to share details about his brother's death with Dr. Bates.) While in high school, he was active on the wrestling team and had a positive relationship with his coach, who helped him stay in school and then get a job when he graduated. Things had been going pretty well when he got laid off. He was particularly proud that he had been helping his girlfriend pay for graduate school, and it is very painful to him that he can no longer help financially support her now.

In contemplating Mr. Franklin's presentation and treatment plan, Dr. Bates has several factors to consider in providing culturally sensitive care. In addition to the other components of an effective evaluation, Dr. Bates might wonder, "What role has discrimination played in Mr. Franklin's current presentation? How does Mr. Franklin conceptualize racism and discrimination in his own experience? How might factors such as Dr. Bates's different race, gender, educational level, and income affect Mr. Franklin's perceptions of her and influence their ability to develop an effective therapeutic relationship? How might Dr. Bates's own values and biases influence her perceptions of Mr. Franklin's problems and their relationship? What might Dr. Bates do to communicate empathy and build a strong therapeutic alliance?"

Culture and the Clinical Assessment

Chronic stress and discrimination based on observable characteristics such as race, ethnicity, and gender are risk factors for poor mental health, as discussed in the section "Discrimination as a Social Determinant of Mental Health." To be complete and to increase diagnostic accuracy, a good clinical assessment will ascertain any potential role of discrimination in the patient's life.

DSM-5 (American Psychiatric Association 2013) has introduced a 16-question Cultural Formulation Interview to be used to improve one's understanding of cultural context in the expression and evaluation of symptoms and dysfunction. Online supplementary modules are also available that focus on explanatory models; level of functioning; social network; psychosocial stressors; spirituality, religion, and moral traditions; cultural identity; coping and help-seeking; and the clinician-patient relationship. When these factors are integrated, the clinician has a context in which to understand the patient's behavior and circumstances.

A cultural formulation describes the individual's cultural and social reference groups and ways in which the cultural context is relevant to clinical care. For example, different risk factors are associated with aspects of different cultures in relation to the development and expression of mental disorders. Religion and family networks also play varied roles as sources of social support, which are potential protective factors that interact with an individual's strengths and coping capacities in shaping clinical presentations. DSM-5 encourages clinicians to assess cultural and contextual features of clinical problems (Lewis-Fernández and Aggarwal 2013). Culture should be broadly defined to take into account any of the patient's individual identities (not only race, ethnicity, and gender but also religion, sexual identity, disability, etc.). Additionally, assessment of cultural context should take into account social and environmental factors such as socioeconomic status and living conditions. These factors may be sources of stress because they interact with an individual's strengths and weaknesses, all of which can serve as sources of resilience as well as challenges.

Understanding cultural reference groups and the meaning and perceived severity of an individual's symptoms within his or her reference group's framework is essential to achieve full understanding of a clinical presentation. What are the idioms of distress through which symptoms or needs for social support are communicated? Cultural factors shape whether a woman will talk to her friends, her doctor, or her pastor about feeling depressed or whether a man will show up at a bar and order a beer rather than admit to himself, let alone to anyone else, that he is feeling depressed. In a cultural milieu that emphasizes certain ideals of masculinity, a man may more readily describe a recent increase in drinking than talk about sadness or depression. Many men may not talk openly about mental health concerns because of cultural stigma attached to mental illnesses. For black men, for example, clinicians may need to consider other expressions of distress, such as withdrawal from friends and family (Neighbors et al. 2012; Watkins et al. 2013).

Attention to cultural and contextual factors is critical because of the ways such factors can contribute to misdiagnosis by clinicians who are not culturally attuned. For example, the diagnosis of depression in black men can be complicated by expressions of mistrust of the clinician as well as mistrust of the world outside the clinic. Such mistrust can be interpreted as paranoia, perhaps leading a clinician's thinking to shift from depressive or mood disorders to psychotic disorders, when historical, structural, and situational contexts shape the ways in which the individual relates to the world and the evaluation process (Watkins and Neighbors 2012; Whaley 1998). In fact, evidence indicates that clinicians overdiagnose schizophrenia among black persons with bipolar disorder, perhaps because cultural differences influence the interpersonal process between patient and clinician, leading to less adequate elicitation of actual symptoms (Gara et al. 2012). Lack of cultural awareness can lead to misdiagnosis and inappropriate treatment (e.g., prescribing antipsychotic medications when antidepressants or mood stabilizers would be clinically indicated). The ways cultural factors may shape the relationship between patient and clinician extend beyond the diagnostic phase as well, shaping the evolution of trust and ability to develop a therapeutic relationship, with potential for a long-lasting impact on treatment outcomes.

Assessing the Effects of Chronic Stress and Discrimination

The impact of chronic stress, including exposure to discrimination, on the development, course, and treatment of poor mental health and mental illnesses has been extensively documented. However, patients may not spontaneously discuss such experiences, especially with a person from a different cultural background. A thorough clinical assessment should include specific probing for chronic stressors and experiences of acute/major and chronic/everyday discrimination that may have contributed to the clinical presentation. This inquiry should include an inventory and appraisal of past and present traumatic events and major stressors in the individual's life, as well as past and current family life and history, immigration history, health history, early losses, and relationship problems, with sensitivity to the ways in which discrimination based on race, ethnicity, sex, gender identity, or other factors can shape all of these. Cultural sensitivity skills are essential to the development of sufficient trust to elicit frank discussion of discriminatory experiences. Such sensitivity should extend to an understanding of institutional racism because so much unfair treatment takes place without intention or knowledge when routine practices advantage one group and marginalize another (Tyrer 2005). Also of concern are daily "microaggressions" (e.g., people crossing the street to keep distance) that have an impact on emotional well-being. Full sensitivity requires understanding that discrimination can be blunt and direct, subtle and hidden, or pervasive and institutionalized.

Clinicians can address discrimination and related risk factors by asking questions, listening carefully and empathically, and showing understanding and support regarding these sources of stress. By recognizing and validating the burden these factors impose, clinicians can deepen the therapeutic relationship and the likelihood that patients will trust them enough to be open and to stay in treatment. Patients who have experienced discrimination—or who come from a different racial or ethnic, educational, socioeconomic, gender, sexual orientation, or religious background—may come to treatment with a sense that the clinician might not be able to relate. Clinicians from privileged backgrounds might not be familiar with the still-prevalent discrimination that exists. Inadequate inquiry can create missed opportunities for alliance building and can contribute to diagnostic errors, inappropriate treatment, or failed therapeutic relationships.

Cultural competency training can help clinicians ask the right questions and improve their ability to listen effectively. Clinicians need to know how to ask the critical questions and to hear and follow up on comments that suggest that deeper feelings exist and need to be explored. This training should also include education about specific culture-bound syndromes and alternative expressions of symptoms and distress (Lewis-Fernández and Aggarwal 2013). For example, as mentioned in the section "Culture and the Clinical Assessment," African American men may be raised with particular notions about masculinity and with awareness of community stigma about mental health issues, making it difficult for them to endorse standard symptoms of depression. Other types of queries may be needed. Clinicians may probe less effectively for depressive symptoms in African Americans because prevalence is lower in blacks than whites, but this may carry greater risk because depression is associated with an increased disease burden and persistence in black populations (Williams et al. 2007). The increased persistence may be due to reduced help-seeking, diagnostic errors, or poor adherence to appropriately prescribed treatments. Clinicians need to be aware that historic maltreatment may have increased reservations among blacks about taking medications; sensitivity to these concerns may improve adherence to treatment recommendations.

Awareness of diversity within racial groups is also needed. Research findings show, for example, that although there are important commonalities in various racial and ethnic experiences, there is also considerable ethnic variation (for example, in major depressive disorder prevalence rates) within the major minority populations (e.g., Caribbean and African American blacks; Vietnamese, Filipino, and Chinese Asian Americans; and Mexican, Puerto Rican, and Cuban subgroups) (Jackson et al. 2011). Findings suggest the need to consider the intersection of factors such as immigration history and gender in addition to race and ethnicity when assessing mood disorders in diverse populations. These factors interact with race and ethnicity, producing heterogeneity within groups. Sweeping generalizations about individuals within a specific racial or ethnic group can be as misleading as generalizations about specific racial or ethnic groups.

For those patients who feel it is important, matching the race (or other identity characteristics) of the clinician with that of the patient might enhance patient comfort and sense of trust. Group therapy programs may also be helpful when they can provide supportive and safe environments for individuals to be with others of similar backgrounds or experiences (Franklin 1997, 1999). Such groups can address shared characteristics that make participants different from others, which may then make it easier for group members to use (or adapt where appropriate) evidence-based treatments that might otherwise be resisted. Such groups can also incorporate standard techniques to more effectively manage the stressors that minority groups experience in greater volume and intensity than others (e.g., by suggesting regular exercise, healthy eating, adequate sleep, meditation, and cultivation of effective support systems).

In 2001, the surgeon general's supplemental report *Mental Health: Culture, Race, and Ethnicity* emphasized that "stigma is a major obstacle preventing people from getting help," reminding us that having a mental disorder can itself make someone a target for discrimination (U.S. Department of Health and Human Services 2001, p. 4). Although the majority of people with mental illnesses, regardless of race or ethnicity, do not receive treatment, minorities have even less availability of and access to mental health care. In addition, minorities often receive a poorer quality of care and are underrepresented in mental health research. Minorities with mental illnesses often have to contend with *double discrimination*, in which individuals experience discrimination both as a racial minority and as a person with a mental illness (Byrne 2000).

Finally, in order to address discrimination, clinicians need to examine their own attitudes, behaviors, and biases. To decrease the potential to engage in discrimination—overt or unintended—individuals need to understand what sustains dominance and exclusion across contexts. The concept of *cultural humility*, which incorporates a commitment to self-evaluation and self-critique to redress power imbalances in the physician-patient dynamic, is a useful reminder that providing culturally sensitive care involves ongoing attention to both the clinician and the patient (Tervalon and Murray-García 1998). Progress has been made, but there is more to be done to challenge and reduce the sometimes invisible structural, cultural, and individual processes that keep recreating forms of oppression, disadvantage, and privilege that sustain injustice.

Policy Approaches to Discrimination as a Social Determinant of Mental Health

The major lesson growing out of analyses of the social determinants of mental health is that a one-size-fits-all framework is not appropriate when thinking about policy, programs, and clinical implications. Race, ethnicity, and nativity combine to influence mental health and mental disorders beyond socioeconomic and other demographic factors. It is obvious that a type of stereotyping that treats cultural differences without nuance may be harmful to developing the most effective clinical approaches, policies, and programs for individuals. An intersectional perspective and interpretation—an approach that recognizes variation within single social categories such as race or ethnic groups—is needed to understand how social determinants create their pernicious effects (Jackson et al. 2010).

Local and State Programs Affecting Discrimination

At the state and local levels, opportunities exist to develop policies and procedures for training and education to extend culturally sensitive knowledge about the nature of social determinants. Local and national professional organizations can also play an important role by providing guidelines and strong recommendations for addressing discrimination and bias in treatment. At the state level, support for the establishment of appropriate cultural competence education at all levels, including continuing professional education in psychiatry, psychology, social work, and a wide range of counseling programs, would be helpful.

In some communities (e.g., African American and Hispanic and Latino), cultural institutions such as churches and other faith-based organizations can play significant roles in recognizing and supporting professional training, identifying psychiatric difficulties, and providing routes into treatment.

Federal Policy and Programs Affecting Discrimination

The federal government, notably through the Equal Employment Opportunity Commission (EEOC), is responsible for enforcing a large number of statutes and executive orders related to many types of discrimination, such as discrimination based on age, gender, race or color, income, use of genetic information, sexual identity, national origin, or religion. Beginning in 1963, a large number of legal mandates have been enacted to protect against a wide range of possible discriminatory behaviors in the workplace, housing, and health care, most notably Title VII of the Civil Rights Act of 1964. Earlier, the Equal Pay Act of 1963 was enacted to make sex differences in pay for equal work illegal. In 1967, the Age Discrimination in Employment Act (ADEA) was enacted. Title I of the Americans with Disabilities Act of 1990 (ADA) extended antidiscrimination legislation to the private sector and state and local governments. Sections 102 and 103 of the Civil Rights Act of 1991 amended Title VII and ADEA to permit jury trials for discrimination cases. Sections 501 and 505 of the Rehabilitation Act of 1973 made it illegal to discriminate against persons with disabilities in the federal government. The Genetic Information Nondiscrimination Act of 2008 (GINA) was added to protect Americans against discrimination in health insurance and employment based on potential genetic predispositions to certain diseases.

The most notable legislation and policies to address race and color discrimination have been at the federal level (Jackson 2000). Policies and actions have been much spottier across the 50 states, although in most cases federal law generally supersedes contradictory state policies. However, there are certain areas, such as marriage equality, in which ongoing state battles may result in more general federal law to address the wide range of state policies.

Adequate federal law exists to address race and color discrimination in public accommodations, housing, employment, and health care. The problem today is finding ways to ensure that governments move swiftly and decisively to address complaints, to hold timely hearings, and, if necessary, to move legal cases faster and more actively through the criminal and civil justice system. The historical unequal and tardy enforcement of existing policies at federal and state levels undermines community and citizen confidence in legal mandates. Slow responsiveness to individual and community complaints by government agencies can have deleterious effects on beliefs in fairness and potential legal redress for transgressions among communities of color. Community monitoring boards (e.g., Focus: HOPE in Detroit) and effective oversight by national organizations, such as the American Civil Liberties Union, the National Association for Latino Community Asset Builders, Human Rights First, the Anti-Defamation League, the Civil Rights Project, the Equal Justice Network, the National Council of La Raza, the National Association for the Advancement of Colored People (NAACP), the NAACP Legal Defense Fund, the Urban League, the Center for Political Studies, and the Southern Poverty Law Center, can provide the necessary national and community oversight and effective political pressure to ensure enforcement.

Promoting Equality and Inclusion: A Role for Everyone

Discrimination based on race and color is particularly pernicious. Internalizing feelings of inferiority creates difficult barriers to overcome. Unfortunately, discrimination begins early in life and is exacerbated by stressful environments and significant barriers to upward mobility. Historically discriminated-against groups have proven to be resilient, and communities of color have developed effective programs for combating many forms of discrimination, such as business-community partnerships, faith-based coalitions, and voluntary legal aid societies to assist individuals and families who experience the negative impact of discrimination, but more actions to combat discrimination are needed.

Schools must develop programs that directly address potential discrimination and legal rights and must build awareness of rights and responsibilities in this area. Public service announcements can be used in more effective ways to educate the populace about what is illegal and what remedies exist for discrimination in housing, employment, and public accommodations. Within community organizations and treatment settings, coalitions and governing bodies should reflect and appropriately represent the diversity of the communities they serve. Most important, we must combine research knowledge about the effects and nature of experienced discrimination, especially the nature of chronic stress, with sensitive clinical interventions designed to create resilience and bolster individual and family behaviors to combat discrimination when it occurs.

Finally, we must recognize that combating discrimination is the responsibility of not only those who are discriminated against but also those who discriminate, either through their own actions or through inactions that maintain institutional forms of discrimination. As we have shown in earlier work, discriminatory behaviors negatively affect the well-being of not only victims but also the perpetrators (Jackson and Volckens 1998). Mental health professionals have a responsibility to advocate for nondiscrimination policies and to react and publicly acknowledge when discriminatory acts are observed.

Key Points

- The linked concepts of chronic stress and experienced discrimination represent a useful conceptual lens to understand one potential etiology of poor physical and mental health.

- Clinical programs and clinicians must be sensitive to the nuances of race, color, ethnicity, and nativity, as well as other aspects of individual differences that engender discrimination, in treating behavioral disorders, especially mood and anxiety disorders.

- Cultural competency and cultural humility training are important vehicles for developing knowledge of different cultural practices, awareness of one's own cultural worldview, attitudes toward differences, and the cross-cultural skills that are needed to understand, be respectful of, and be responsive to the needs of diverse patients.

- Adequate antidiscrimination legislation exists, especially at the federal level; what is needed is more effective enforcement of laws and administrative mandates.

- Communities affected by discrimination have to assume greater responsibility in educating and developing effective antiracism and antidiscrimination movements through collaborations with private and government institutions and majority and minority racial communities. Vigorously working to eliminate discrimination is the responsibility of not only those who are discriminated against but also those who might discriminate, either through their own actions or through their inactions that contribute to maintaining institutional forms of discrimination.

References

Alexander M: The New Jim Crow: Mass Incarceration in the Age of Colorblindness. New York, The New Press, 2010

American Psychiatric Association: Diagnostic and Statistical Manual of Mental Disorders, 5th Edition. Arlington, VA, American Psychiatric Association, 2013

Barnes LL, de Leon CF, Lewis TT, et al: Perceived discrimination and mortality in a population-based study of older adults. Am J Public Health 98(7):1241–1247, 2008 18511732

Bobo L, Kluegel JR: Opposition to race-targeting: self-interest, stratification ideology, or racial attitudes? Am Sociol Rev 58:443–464, 1993

Bonilla-Silva E: Rethinking racism: toward a structural interpretation. Am Sociol Rev 62(3):465–480, 1997

Brown TN: Measuring self-perceived racial and ethnic discrimination in social surveys. Sociol Spectr 21(3):377–392, 2001

Brown TN, Williams DR, Jackson JS, et al: "Being black and feeling blue": the mental health consequences of racial discrimination. Race Soc 2:117–131, 2000

Byrne P: Stigma of mental illness and ways of diminishing it. Adv Psychiatr Treat 6:65–72, 2000

Chae DH, Lincoln KD, Adler NE, et al: Do experiences of racial discrimination predict cardiovascular disease among African American men? The moderating role of internalized negative racial group attitudes. Soc Sci Med 71(6):1182–1188, 2010 20659782

Clark R: Perceived racism and vascular reactivity in black college women: moderating effects of seeking social support. Health Psychol 25(1):20–25, 2006 16448294

Clark R, Anderson NB, Clark VR, et al: Racism as a stressor for African Americans. A biopsychosocial model. Am Psychol 54(10):805–816, 1999 10540593

Cogburn CD, Griffin TM, Jackson JS: Race and mental health disparities, in Encyclopedia of Race and Racism, 2nd Edition. Edited by Mason PL. New York, Macmillan Reference, 2013, pp 126–131

Fischer CS, Hout M: Century of Difference: How America Changed in the Last One Hundred Years. New York, Russell Sage Foundation, 2006

Franklin AJ: Friendship issues between African American men in a therapeutic support group. J Afr Am Men 3:29–43, 1997

Franklin AJ: Invisibility syndrome and racial identity development in psychotherapy and counseling African American men. Couns Psychol 27:761–793, 1999

Gara MA, Vega WA, Arndt S, et al: Influence of patient race and ethnicity on clinical assessment in patients with affective disorders. Arch Gen Psychiatry 69(6):593–600, 2012 22309972

Gee GC, Spencer M, Chen J, et al: The association between self-reported racial discrimination and 12-month DSM-IV mental disorders among Asian Americans nationwide. Soc Sci Med 64(10):1984–1996, 2007 17374553

Glaeser E, Vigdor J: The End of the Segregated Century: Racial Separation in America's Neighborhoods, 1890–2010 (Civic Report No 66). New York, Manhattan Institute for Policy Research, 2012

Griffin TM, Jackson JS: Racial differences, in The Corsini Encyclopedia of Psychology, 4th Edition. Edited by Weiner IB, Craighead WE. New York, Wiley, 2009, pp 1411–1413

House JS: Understanding social factors and inequalities in health: 20th century progress and 21st century prospects. J Health Soc Behav 43(2):125–142, 2002 12096695

Jackson JS: New Directions: African Americans in a Diversifying Nation (NPA Report No 297).Washington, DC, National Policy Association and Program for Research on Black Americans, University of Michigan, 2000

Jackson JS, Volckens J: Community stressors and racism: structural and individual perspectives on racial bias, in Addressing Community Problems: Research and Interventions (Applied Social Psychology Annual 265). Edited by Arriaga XB. Thousand Oaks, CA, Sage, 1998, pp 19–51

Jackson JS, Caldwell C, Williams DR, et al: National Survey of American Life, 2001–2003. Ann Arbor, MI, Inter-university Consortium for Political and Social Research, 2001–2003

Jackson JS, Williams DR, Torres M: Discrimination, health and mental health: the social stress process, in Socioeconomic Conditions, Stress and Mental Disorders: Toward a New Synthesis of Research and Public Policy. Edited by Maney A, Ramos J. Bethesda, MD, National Institutes of Health Office of Behavioral and Social Research, 2003, pp 145–178

Jackson JS, Govia IO, Sellers SL: Race and ethnic influences over the life-course, in Handbook of Aging and the Social Sciences, 7th Edition. Edited by Binstock RH, George LK. New York, Academic Press, 2010, pp 91–103

Jackson JS, Abelson JA, Berglund PA, et al: The intersection of race, ethnicity, immigration, and cultural influences on the nature and distribution of mental disorders, in The Conceptual Evolution of DSM-5. Edited by Regier DA, Narrow WE, Kuhl WE, et al. Washington, DC, American Psychiatric Publishing, 2011, pp 267–286

Karlsen S, Nazroo JY: Relation between racial discrimination, social class, and health among ethnic minority groups. Am J Public Health 92(4):624–631, 2002 11919063

Kressin NR, Raymond KL, Manze M: Perceptions of race/ethnicity-based discrimination: a review of measures and evaluation of their usefulness for the health care setting. J Health Care Poor Underserved 19(3):697–730, 2008 18677066

Krieger N: Racial and gender discrimination: risk factors for high blood pressure? Soc Sci Med 30(12):1273–1281, 1990 2367873

Krieger N: Methods for the scientific study of discrimination and health: an ecosocial approach. Am J Public Health 102(5):936–944, 2012 22420803

Krieger N, Sidney S: Racial discrimination and blood pressure: the CARDIA Study of young black and white adults. Am J Public Health 86(10):1370–1378, 1996 8876504

Landrine H, Klonoff EA: The schedule of racist events: a measure of racial discrimination and a study of its negative physical and mental health consequences. J Black Psychol 22:144–168, 1996

LaVeist TA: Why we should continue to study race…but do a better job: an essay on race, racism and health. Ethn Dis 6(1–2):21–29, 1996 8882833

Lazarus RS, Folkman S: Stress, Appraisal, and Coping. New York, Springer, 1984

Levine DS, Himle JA, Abelson JM, et al: Discrimination and social anxiety disorder among African-Americans, Caribbean blacks, and non-Hispanic whites. J Nerv Ment Dis 202(3):224–230, 2014 24566508

Lewis TT, Everson-Rose SA, Powell LH, et al: Chronic exposure to everyday discrimination and coronary artery calcification in African-American women: the SWAN Heart Study. Psychosom Med 68(3):362–368, 2006 16738065

Lewis-Fernández R, Aggarwal NK: Culture and psychiatric diagnosis. Adv Psychosom Med 33:15–30, 2013 23816860

Link BG, Phelan J: Social conditions as fundamental causes of disease. J Health Soc Behav 35(Spec No):80–94, 1995 7560851

Massey DS, Denton NA: American Apartheid: Segregation and the Making of the Underclass, Cambridge, MA, Harvard University Press, 1993

Neighbors HW, Watkins DC, Abelson JM: Man up, man down: adult black men talk about success, disappointment, manhood, and depression. Presented at the American Men's Health Association meeting, Minneapolis, MN, March 2012

Omi M, Winant H: Racial Formation in the United States: From the 1960s to the 1990s. New York, Routledge, 1994

Pager D, Shepherd H: The sociology of discrimination: racial discrimination in employment, housing, credit, and consumer markets. Annu Rev Sociol 34:181–209, 2008 20689680

Pascoe EA, Smart Richman L: Perceived discrimination and health: a meta-analytic review. Psychol Bull 135(4):531–554, 2009 19586161

Pearlin LI: The sociological study of stress. J Health Soc Behav 30(3):241–256, 1989 2674272

Phelan JC, Link BG, Tehranifar P: Social conditions as fundamental causes of health inequalities: theory, evidence, and policy implications. J Health Soc Behav 51(suppl):S28–S40, 2010 20943581

Richman LS, Bennett GG, Pek J, et al: Discrimination, dispositions, and cardiovascular responses to stress. Health Psychol 26(6):675–683, 2007 18020838

Ryan AM, Gee GC, Laflamme DF: The association between self-reported discrimination, physical health and blood pressure: findings from African Americans, Black immigrants, and Latino immigrants in New Hampshire. J Health Care Poor Underserved 17(2)(suppl):116–132, 2006 16809879

Schuman H, Krysan M, Steeh C, et al: Racial Attitudes in America: Trends and Interpretations. Cambridge, MA, Harvard University Press, 1997

Selye H: The Stress of Life. New York, McGraw-Hill, 1956

Soto JA, Dawson-Andoh NA, BeLue R: The relationship between perceived discrimination and generalized anxiety disorder among African Americans, Afro Caribbeans, and non-Hispanic whites. J Anxiety Disord 25(2):258–265, 2011 21041059

Telles EE: Race in Another America: The Significance of Skin Color in Brazil. Princeton, NJ, Princeton University Press, 2004

Tervalon M, Murray-García J: Cultural humility versus cultural competence: a critical distinction in defining physician training outcomes in multicultural education. J Health Care Poor Underserved 9(2):117–125, 1998 10073197

Tyrer P: Combating editorial racism in psychiatric publications. Br J Psychiatry 186:1–3, 2005 15630115

U.S. Department of Health and Human Services: Mental Health: Culture, Race, and Ethnicity—A Supplement to Mental Health: A Report of the Surgeon General. Rockville, MD, Substance Abuse and Mental Health Services Administration, 2001

Watkins DC, Neighbors HW: Social determinants of depression and the black male experience, in Social Determinants of Health Among African-American Men. Edited by Treadwell HM, Xanthos C, Holden KB. San Francisco, CA, Jossey-Bass, 2012, pp 39–62

Watkins DC, Abelson JM, Jefferson SO: "Their depression is something different...it would have to be": findings from a qualitative study of black women's perceptions of depression in black men. Am J Men Health 7(4)(suppl):45S–57S, 2013 23784520

Whaley AL: Black psychiatric patients' reactions to the cultural mistrust inventory. J Natl Med Assoc 90(12):776–778, 1998 9884498

Williams DR, Mohammed SA: Discrimination and racial disparities in health: evidence and needed research. J Behav Med 32(1):20–47, 2009 19030981

Williams DR, Yan Yu, Jackson JS, Anderson NB: Racial differences in physical and mental health: socio-economic status, stress and discrimination. J Health Psychol 2(3):335–351, 1997 22013026

Williams DR, Neighbors HW, Jackson JS: Racial/ethnic discrimination and health: findings from community studies. Am J Public Health 93(2):200–208, 2003 12554570

Williams DR, González HM, Neighbors H, et al: Prevalence and distribution of major depressive disorder in African Americans, Caribbean blacks, and non-Hispanic whites: results from the National Survey of American Life. Arch Gen Psychiatry 64(3):305–315, 2007 17339519

Williams DR, Haile R, Mohammed SA, et al: Perceived discrimination and psychological well-being in the U.S.A. and South Africa. Ethn Health 17(1-2):111–133, 2012a 22339224

Williams DR, John DA, Oyserman D, et al: Research on discrimination and health: an exploratory study of unresolved conceptual and measurement issues. Am J Public Health 102(5):975–978, 2012b 22420798

3

Adverse Early Life Experiences

Carol Koplan, M.D.
Anna Chard, M.P.H.

The Child is father of the Man.

William Wordsworth, 1770–1850, in "The Rainbow"

Influenced by Freud's late nineteenth and early twentieth century theories about the role of childhood experiences and the impact of trauma on the development of adult neuroses, scientists, researchers, and mental health professionals began to explore the relationship of early childhood experiences to adult mental health outcomes. More recently, epidemiological studies demonstrated the widespread prevalence of adverse early life experiences (AELEs) and the significant associations between these experiences and a variety of later negative mental health outcomes (Anda et al. 2002; Dube et al. 2001, 2003; Norman et al. 2012; Whitfield et al. 2005). In addition, researchers described physiological mechanisms by which childhood stress can alter the developing brain, thus leading to risky behaviors, poor mental health, and mental disorders (National Scientific Council on the Developing Child 2005, 2010). Furthermore, evidence now shows that AELEs in utero and from birth through age 18 can lead to negative mental health outcomes throughout the life span (Allen et al. 1998; Lou et al. 1994; Philipps and O'Hara 1991). Prevention science has shown that improving malleable adverse social relationships of young individuals within their families, neighborhoods, schools, and overall environment can prevent or reverse subsequent negative outcomes in adolescence and adulthood (National Scientific Council on the Developing Child 2005, 2010). Moreover, interventions targeting individuals, families, institutions, and society as a whole can moderate these outcomes to improve the physical and mental health of children, the adults they become, and the next generation.

Adverse Early Life Experiences: An Overview

Definition of Adverse Early Life Experiences

AELEs are inconsistent, stressful, threatening, hurtful, traumatic, or neglectful social interchanges experienced by fetuses, infants, children, or adolescents. These interchanges occur between the developing child and individuals around him or her in caretaking, school, or neighborhood environments and are risk factors for long-term physical and mental health consequences. AELEs also encompass a wide range of circumstances, such as poverty, hunger, inequality, and discrimination, although these broader effects are difficult to address without major societal changes. AELEs associated with problematic social relationships are often malleable and thus can be reduced with clinical or public health interventions as well as local, state, and federal policies that promote safe, stable, and nurturing environments. In this chapter we focus on traumatic or otherwise adverse relationships and experiences that occur where children develop, live, learn, and play and how they can affect both mental health and the risk for mental disorders.

Prevalence of Adverse Early Life Experiences in the United States

In the 1980s and 1990s, Dr. Vincent Felitti recognized that many individuals who were morbidly obese in his health maintenance organization (HMO) clinic responded only partially to treatment for their obesity. During their treatment, some of these patients revealed that they had experienced abuse and other childhood adversities. Dr. Robert Anda, an epidemiologist from the Centers for Disease Control and Prevention (CDC), was struck by a presentation of these findings at a national meeting in 1990. This presentation catalyzed a collaboration between Felitti and Anda and their respective organizations to explore the prevalence of early childhood adversities among a middle-class, HMO-insured population and simultaneously to review this population's health outcomes (Corwin 2012).

In 1998, this team of researchers published their findings in a groundbreaking study called the Adverse Childhood Experiences Study (ACE Study) (Felitti et al. 1998). This retrospective study surveyed 17,000 patients (average age 57) about three types of abuse (physical, sexual, and emotional), two types of neglect (physical and emotional), and five types of family dysfunction (parents separated or divorced, household member with an alcohol or a drug use disorder, household member with a mental illness, household member incarcerated, and household member involved in intimate partner violence) that they had experienced as children. An affirmative response to a particular experience was assigned 1 point, creating an adverse childhood experiences (ACEs) score ranging from 0 to 10. As shown in Figure 3–1, ACEs were found to be highly prevalent, with 63.6% of the population reporting one or more ACEs (Felitti and Anda 2010; Dube et al. 2001).

A decade later, the CDC organized surveys of two additional, more representative samples of adults. Using the Behavioral Risk Factor Surveillance System (BRFSS), researchers conducted surveys on eight ACEs (with the two neglect questions from the original ACE Study being excluded) in 5 states in 2009 (Bynum et al. 2010) and 10 states and the District of Columbia in 2010 (Gilbert 2013). These studies corroborated the widespread prevalence of ACEs in the U.S. population (see Figure 3–2).

Studies on AELEs are not limited to the ACE Study and its substudies (more than 60 publications to date) (Centers for Disease Control and Prevention 2013b). For example, a national survey of adolescents and the caretakers of children was performed in 2008 (Finkelhor et al. 2009). This survey had the advantage of a shorter interval between childhood events and the survey, thus reducing the impact of recall error. Furthermore, this survey differed from the ACE Study because it cataloged both indirect and direct exposures to violence. Indirect violence involved hearing about violence targeted toward a family member or friend, whereas direct violence was experienced by the child or adolescent himself or herself. In the year prior to the survey, 60% of these young people had been exposed to violence: 50% were assaulted at least once, 25% witnessed a violent act, 10% saw interpersonal violence among family members, and 10% reported experiencing child maltreatment (Finkelhor et al. 2009). Thus, although this particular study measured different domains of AELEs than the ACE Study, the results confirmed the high prevalence of AELEs in the U.S. population.

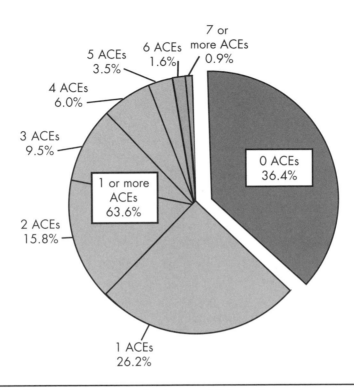

FIGURE 3–1. Prevalence of adverse childhood experiences (ACEs) among U.S. adults.

Source. Dube et al. 2001.

The widespread prevalence of AELEs in the United States is further supported by the number of cases of suspected child maltreatment reported to state protective agencies. In 2011, reports of abuse and neglect were filed on behalf of 3,000,000 children. Following investigations, reports for 681,000 of these children were substantiated (U.S. Department of Health and Human Services 2012). Many victims of confirmed child abuse are placed in foster care, where they are susceptible to further separations, instability, and even additional trauma. In 2011 alone, 400,540 children in the United States were living in foster care (Child Welfare Information Gateway 2013a). Other populations of children vulnerable to AELEs are those who are homeless (1,600,000 in 2010) (National Center on Family Homelessness 2011), those who are refugees, those in juvenile detention, and those in war zones or postdisaster settings. In these environments, not only are children and adolescents living under very

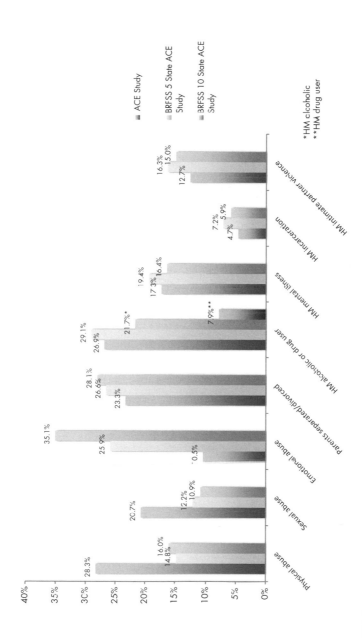

FIGURE 3–2. Results from three studies measuring adverse childhood experience (ACE) prevalence in the United States.

BRFSS=Behavioral Risk Factor Surveillance System; HM=household member.
Source. Data from Dube et al. 2001; Bynum et al. 2010; Gilbert 2013.

stressful and traumatic circumstances but often so are their caretakers, thus exacerbating the overall impact of AELEs.

Whereas maltreatment is characterized by hurtful actions perpetrated by adults toward children and adolescents, bullying is an AELE perpetrated by young people toward those in their same age group. In the past, people regarded bullying as a normal part of growing up (Olweus 1994). However, researchers have elaborated on the associations between bullying and negative mental health outcomes (Arseneault et al. 2006; Sourander et al. 2007), thus recognizing bullying as an AELE with serious repercussions. Bullying is widespread (Limber et al. 2013) and often occurs in schools, involving a real or perceived imbalance of power between bullies and victims, with harmful actions repeated over time. Similar to the range of types of maltreatment that a parent or caretaker may perpetrate against a child, bullying may be perpetrated verbally, physically, and emotionally (Centers for Disease Control and Prevention 2012). Moreover, with advancements in technology, bullying has also moved beyond the playground to texting and social media on the Internet (cyberbullying) (Centers for Disease Control and Prevention 2012; Limber et al. 2013).

Surveys of children and adolescents in the United States have demonstrated that a significant number of children between the third and twelfth grades are involved in some way with bullying (19.6%), with the highest incidence of bullying occurring in elementary school and decreasing with increasing grade level. Thirteen percent of students report being a victim of bullying, 4% are perpetrators of bullying, and 3% are both perpetrators and victims, known as *bully-victims* (Limber et al. 2013). Lesbian and gay youth are more vulnerable to bullying than their non–sexual minority peers; a survey of Oregon teens revealed that 60.2% of lesbian and gay youth reported being victimized in the 30 days prior to the survey compared with 28.8% of their heterosexual counterparts (Hatzenbuehler and Keyes 2013). These statistics are notable because they demonstrate that many children and adolescents in the United States are subjected to the AELE of bullying outside of their home environment, with an even larger proportion of minority and vulnerable populations experiencing bullying.

Adverse Early Life Experiences as Social Determinants of Health

AELEs are social determinants of health—they are traumatic, stressful, harmful, or neglectful conditions in young people's social and physical environments that are shaped by social circumstances and that negatively impact health. These social determinants are the result of an array of complex interrelated factors involving individual, familial, organizational, and societal characteristics related to how people spend their daily lives.

ACE Study researchers have visually conceptualized ACEs as a determinant of physical, mental, and behavioral health outcomes in the ACE Study Pyramid (Centers for Disease Control and Prevention 2013a) (Figure 3–3). This model illustrates the progression from ACEs to adolescent risk behaviors; to adult disease, disability, and social problems; and, finally, to premature death. The arrows indicate gaps in knowledge about the progression from one stage to the next, representing important opportunities for scientific inquiry (Centers for Disease Control and Prevention 2013a).

Risk factors, referred to as "adoption of health-risk behaviors" on the ACE Study Pyramid, such as smoking and substance use disorders, are traditionally seen as underlying factors for most chronic diseases. The ACE Study researchers explain that these behavioral risks often begin as a result of adolescents coping with chronic stress, which stems from early childhood trauma. In a study examining the relationship between ACEs and ischemic heart disease, researchers found that not only did risk increase as one's ACE score increased but also a graded relationship existed between one's ACE score and more proximal risk factors, such as smoking, physical inactivity, and severe obesity (Dong et al. 2004). Some risk factors are efforts at "self-medication" through the use of substances such as nicotine or alcohol that provide psychoactive benefits (Felitti and Anda 2010). This finding is significant in demonstrating that AELEs precede the development of many traditionally accepted risk factors for chronic disease; thus, recognition of this association opens the door for more robust chronic disease prevention research and activities.

The ACE Study and its subsequent substudies have provided strong evidence implicating childhood abuse, neglect, and family dysfunction as social determinants in a child's environment that lead to negative physical health and mental health outcomes throughout the life span. Additionally, these studies are suggestive of a *dose-response relationship*, where the risk for chronic conditions, such as ischemic heart disease, cancer, chronic obstructive pulmonary disease, autoimmune diseases, hepatitis or jaundice, and skeletal fractures, increases in a graded fashion as one's ACE score increases (Anda et al. 2008; Dong et al. 2004; Dube et al. 2009; Felitti and Anda 2010). Furthermore, research by

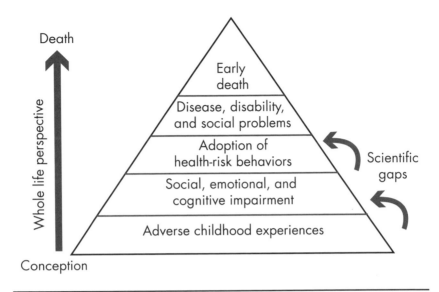

FIGURE 3–3.   ACE Study Pyramid.

Source.   Centers for Disease Control and Prevention: Adverse Childhood Experiences Study Pyramid. Atlanta, GA, Centers for Disease Control and Prevention, January 18, 2013. Available at: http://www.cdc.gov/ace/pyramid.htm. Accessed June 24, 2013.

Brown et al. (2009) showed that adults experiencing six or more ACEs had significantly shorter life spans compared with adults experiencing no ACEs. Although the relationship between one's ACE score and life span was not significant after controlling for traditional risk factors for shorter life expectancy, these traditional risk factors in and of themselves are often attributable to underlying ACE-related health and social determinants. Additional research investigating the association between AELEs and life span is warranted.

Health outcomes associated with AELEs represent a significant burden of chronic conditions in the U.S. population. In addition to the ACE Study, several other studies have confirmed an association between childhood trauma, abuse, and neglect and poor physical health in adulthood in diverse populations (Draper et al. 2008; Rich-Edwards et al. 2010; Walker et al. 1999; Widom et al. 2012). These studies emphasize the impact of AELEs as an underlying cause of chronic physical diseases; however, in this chapter we now focus on the impact of AELEs as underlying causes of poor mental health throughout the life span.

Adverse Early Life Experiences as Social Determinants of Mental Health

Traumatic experiences in a child's social environment that result in negative physical health outcomes are similarly associated with negative mental health outcomes. Indeed, the links between AELEs and risk for negative mental health outcomes in adulthood are well documented (Anda et al. 2002; Dube et al. 2001, 2003; Whitfield et al. 2005). Follow-up research of the original ACE Study found that certain ACEs and combinations of ACEs are risk factors for a host of mental and behavioral disorders, such as depression, problematic alcohol use, illicit drug use, hallucinations, and suicide attempts (Table 3–1) (Anda et al. 2002; Dube et al. 2001, 2003; Whitfield et al. 2005). Furthermore, as shown in Figure 3–4, a combination of several ACEs involving violent exposures during childhood increases the risk for becoming a victim or perpetrator of violence as an adult (Whitfield et al. 2003), thus perpetuating the cycle of violence across generations.

Additionally, ACEs have a cumulative effect on mental health, in which an increasing ACE score is positively correlated with an increased risk for experiencing numerous poor mental health outcomes. Although many epidemiological studies have shown that the risk for most mental disorders increases in a graded fashion as one's ACE score increases (Felitti et al. 1998), a later study demonstrated that the lifetime risk for suicide attempts increases exponentially as one's ACE score increases (Dube et al. 2001). For example, the risk of lifetime suicide attempts for adults who reported four, five, six, or seven or more ACEs was 3.8, 11.2, 13.2, and 29.8 times higher, respectively, than for adults reporting no ACEs (Dube et al. 2001). This strong association points to the need for interventions targeted at preventing AELEs to decrease suicidality in the U.S. population.

The relationship between several of the maltreatment-related ACEs and poor mental health outcomes was further corroborated in a meta-analysis reviewing 124 studies in predominantly high-income countries (Norman et al. 2012). The analysis found that physical abuse, emotional abuse, and neglect were all significantly associated with a range of poor mental health outcomes, including depressive and anxiety disorders, drug abuse, eating disorders, and suicidal behaviors, as well as risky sexual behaviors and sexually transmitted infections. Furthermore, much like the ACE Study, the analysis highlighted a dose-response relationship between many AELEs and mental health outcomes. For exam-

TABLE 3–1.   Associations between adverse childhood experiences and mental health outcomes

	Depression[a]	Alcoholism[a]	Illicit drug use[b]	Hallucinations[c]	Attempted suicide[d]
Physical abuse	1.9 (1.7–2.1)	1.9 (1.6–2.3)	2.0 (1.8–2.3)	1.7 (1.4–2.1)	3.4 (2.9–4.0)
Sexual abuse	1.7 (1.5–2.0)	1.9 (1.6–2.4)	2.0 (1.8–2.3)	1.7 (1.4–2.1)	3.4 (2.9–4.0)
Emotional abuse	2.7 (2.3–3.1)	2.9 (2.3–3.6)	2.1 (1.7–2.5)	2.3 (1.8–3.0)	5.0 (4.2–5.9)
Parents separated/divorced	1.3 (1.2–1.5)	1.7 (1.4–2.1)	1.7 (1.5–1.9)	1.3 (1.1–1.6)	1.9 (1.6–2.2)
HM alcoholic or drug user	1.6 (1.3–2.0)	1.7 (1.2–2.4)	2.1 (1.8–2.4)	1.4 (1.1–1.8)	2.1 (1.8–2.5)
HM with a mental illness	2.5 (2.2–2.8)	2.0 (1.6–2.5)	1.9 (1.7–2.2)	2.5 (2.0–3.1)	3.3 (2.8–3.9)
HM incarceration	1.4 (1.1–1.8)	2.1 (1.4–3.0)	1.9 (1.5–2.4)	1.2 (0.8–1.9)	2.5 (2.0–3.2)
HM intimate partner violence	1.9 (1.6–2.1)	2.5 (2.0–3.1)	1.6 (1.4–1.9)	1.5 (1.1–2.0)	2.6 (2.2–3.1)

TABLE 3–1. Associations between adverse childhood experiences and mental health outcomes *(continued)*

	Depression[a]	Alcoholism[a]	Illicit drug use[b]	Hallucinations[c]	Attempted suicide[d]
Physical neglect[e]	—	—	1.3 (1.1–1.6)	—	—
Emotional neglect[e]	—	—	1.8 (1.6–2.1)	—	—

Note. Values are adjusted odds ratios, with 95% confidence intervals given in parentheses. Dashes represent domains not measured in select studies. HM=household member.
[a]Data from only ACE Study wave 1 (*n*=9,346) (Anda et al. 2002).
[b]Data from only ACE Study wave 2 (*n*=8,613) (Dube et al. 2003).
[c]Data from both waves of the ACE Study (*n*=17,337) (Whitfield et al. 2001).
[d]Data from both waves of the ACE Study (*n*=17,337) (Dube et al. 2005).
[e]Questions included in ACE Study wave 2 (*n*=8,613).

The Social Determinants of Mental Health

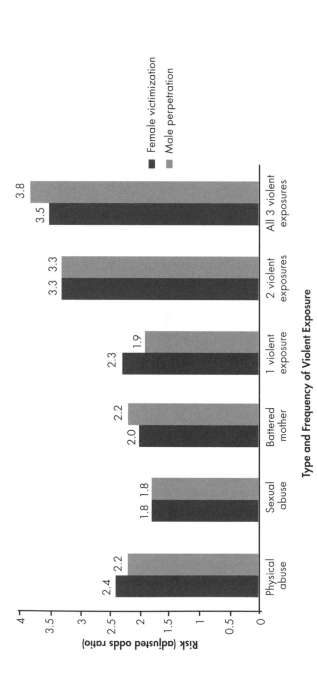

FIGURE 3-4. Association between exposure to violence as a child and risk of being a victim or perpetrator of interpersonal violence as an adult.

Source. Whitfield et al. 2001.

ple, anxiety disorders were more likely among those who experienced frequent physical abuse, and depressive disorders were more likely among those who experienced frequent neglect compared with those who experienced physical abuse or neglect only occasionally. Additionally, this review was particularly significant because unlike the ACE Study, which was retrospective, it included 16 prospective studies. Because the meta-analysis examined research conducted in more than 18 countries, it demonstrated that AELEs are a worldwide concern (Norman et al. 2012).

Adverse Experiences in the Prenatal Period, Infancy, and Early Childhood

Stress experienced by the fetus and the infant may also be classified as an AELE and thus may be considered a social determinant that can lead to negative mental health outcomes. There are three main pathways through which maternal stress may affect the fetus: 1) maternal behaviors (such as engaging in substance abuse), 2) depriving the fetus of oxygen and nutrients through reduction in blood flow, and 3) transporting stress-related hormones to the fetus through the placenta (DiPietro 2004). Normal fetal maturation and the birth process rely on some stress-related hormones, such as cortisol. However, variations in these hormones, especially early in pregnancy, may lead to alterations in the fetus's stress response system (Huizink et al. 2004). The role of prenatal maternal stress on child development has been well documented in the scientific literature. Maternal stress during pregnancy has been linked to preterm birth, low birth weight (Copper et al. 1996), and smaller head size at birth (Lou et al. 1994). These physical health outcomes can be related to later cognitive outcomes, such as lower intelligence quotient (IQ) (Gale et al. 2006; Hack et al. 1995). Additionally, studies demonstrate an association between maternal emotional difficulties during pregnancy and disruptive behavior disorders in infants (Allen et al. 1998). Similarly, maternal exposure to major stressors, such as war, has been associated with children experiencing delayed motor development, antisocial behavior, and an increased incidence of behavioral problems (Meijer 1985).

The mental, social, and behavioral health of children and adolescents is also impacted by AELEs occurring after birth. Between 10% and 15% of mothers suffer from postpartum depression (O'Hara and Swain 1996). Children of mothers experiencing postpartum depression are at risk for a multitude of adverse outcomes, including poor cognitive functioning

(Hay et al. 2001), behavioral disturbances, and antisocial behavior (Murray et al. 1999), although findings are mixed (Philipps and O'Hara 1991). Women who experience postpartum depression have a significantly higher risk of subsequent episodes of depression (Philipps and O'Hara 1991). Thus, the presence of a mother's recurring or persistent symptoms of depression beyond the postpartum period may be what is associated with an increased risk of long-term mental health problems among her children (Agnafors et al. 2013; Philipps and O'Hara 1991). Additionally, research points to the timing of first exposure to maternal depression as a significant risk factor in the development of emotional disorders among children (Naicker et al. 2012). A study in Canada found no association between a child's initial exposure to maternal depression during the postpartum period and an emotional disorder in adolescence; however, children whose initial exposure to maternal depression occurred between ages 2 and 3 or between ages 4 and 5 were almost twice as likely to experience an emotional disorder in adolescence compared with their counterparts not exposed to maternal depression (Naicker et al. 2012). The convergence of this research indicates that mothers and expectant mothers who have demonstrated a risk for depression should be targeted for intervention programs early in pregnancy, with continued monitoring throughout the early lives of their children to prevent or reduce recurring depression.

Bullying as an Adverse Early Life Experience Affecting Mental Health

AELEs also occur outside of the home, for example, in schools. In recent years, concerns surrounding young people's involvement in bullying have grown because incidents of children injuring or killing themselves or others have been in media headlines. Unfortunately, this phenomenon of bullying and its negative consequences are not isolated circumstances. A preponderance of research has demonstrated that children who are involved in bullying—as victims, as perpetrators, or as both—manifest a range of poor mental health outcomes in childhood, adolescence, and adulthood, including self-harm behaviors, anxiety disorders, and antisocial personality disorder (Arseneault et al. 2006; Sourander et al. 2007).

Prospective, longitudinal research on mental health outcomes of bullying has found significantly more internalizing problems (defined as self-harming behaviors), unhappiness at school (Arseneault et al. 2006), and occurrences of generalized anxiety disorder (Sourander et al.

2007) among children who were victims of bullying compared with children who were not bullied. However, victims of bullying are not the only group for whom bullying has a deleterious effect. Perpetrators of bullying are significantly more likely to be diagnosed with antisocial personality disorder in adulthood (Sourander et al. 2007). Furthermore, children who are bully-victims have significantly more internalizing problems and externalizing problems (defined as harmful behaviors toward others), fewer prosocial behaviors (i.e., voluntary behaviors benefiting others), more unhappiness, and greater academic difficulty than both those who are only victims of bullying and those who are not bullied (Arseneault et al. 2006). Also, bully-victims are significantly more likely to be diagnosed with both generalized anxiety disorder and antisocial personality disorder in adulthood (Sourander et al. 2007). Thus, children who are bully-victims are distinct from victims who do not also perpetrate bullying and demonstrate even more pervasive and severe negative mental health outcomes associated with bullying. Furthermore, these mental health manifestations occur independently of other risk factors contributing to poor mental health in the lives of bullies, victims, and bully-victims, indicating that involvement in bullying is an AELE that uniquely contributes to poor mental health (Arseneault et al. 2006; Sourander et al. 2007).

Another negative mental health outcome of bullying that causes great concern is suicidal behavior, which encompasses suicide, suicide attempts, and suicidal ideation. A review of 31 studies examining the associations between bullying and suicidal behavior found that the risk of suicidal behavior was up to 11 times greater among adolescents involved in bullying compared with adolescent counterparts who were not (Brunstein Klomek et al. 2010). Furthermore, the associations between bullying and suicidal behavior exist after controlling for other risk factors for suicide, such as depression (Borowsky et al. 2013; Brunstein Klomek et al. 2010), indicating that bullying is an independent risk factor for suicidal behavior. However, research suggests that the association between involvement in bullying and suicidal behavior may be more prominent in the context of comorbid mental health issues (Brunstein Klomek et al. 2010), which may have serious implications for adolescents experiencing additional AELEs. Moreover, bully-victims demonstrate the greatest risk for persistent suicidality (Borowsky et al. 2013; Brunstein Klomek et al. 2010), supporting other research findings that bully-victims suffer the greatest negative mental health effects as a result of bullying involvement (Arseneault et al. 2006; Sourander et al. 2007).

Mechanisms Linking Adverse Early Life Experiences to Mental Health Outcomes

In the past two decades, research has begun to delineate the mechanisms that lead from AELEs to mental health outcomes throughout the life span, as illustrated in the ACE Study Pyramid. Researchers have been focusing on how the stress caused by AELEs can affect biological systems in the developing child. The body's stress response is initiated and maintained by three major brain circuits: the locus coeruleus–norepinephrine system, the extrahypothalamic corticotropin-releasing factor system, and the hypothalamic-pituitary-adrenal axis (cortisol) system (LaPrairie et al. 2010). These systems are especially malleable during the prenatal and early childhood periods, meaning that stressful experiences during these times may shape how easily these neural circuits are activated, as well as how readily they may be turned off (National Scientific Council on the Developing Child 2005). Activations of these brain systems in response to acute threats are generally beneficial because they help individuals adjust homeostasis and react to potential threats (LaPrairie et al. 2010). However, prolonged activation of these systems because of chronic stress, also referred to as *toxic stress* (National Scientific Council on the Developing Child 2005), can cause alterations in the brain development of children (LaPrairie et al. 2010; Middlebrooks and Audage 2008) and can ultimately lead to cognitive deficits, a lower threshold for tolerance of stressful events (National Scientific Council on the Developing Child 2005), dysfunction, and maladaptation (LaPrairie et al. 2010).

A series of monographs reported findings about the effects of toxic stress on the genetic structures of fetuses, infants, and children, as well as the mental and behavioral outcomes of genetic alterations (National Scientific Council on the Developing Child 2005, 2010). The relatively recent field of epigenetics has shown that many noninherited environmental factors and experiences have the ability to chemically mark genes and control their functions (National Scientific Council on the Developing Child 2010), thus creating a new genetic landscape, or epigenome. These environmentally induced genes can cause temporary gene expression or enduring gene expression, which can transfer to the next generation. Additionally, altering the epigenome can influence how well or how poorly one responds to stress; those with poor stress responses can be epigenetically predisposed to depressive and anxiety disorders. However, although the epigenetic modifications linked to these outcomes were once thought to be permanent, research suggests that there are interventions that may reverse the deoxyribonucleic acid (DNA) changes caused by toxic stress (National Scientific Council on the Developing Child 2010). This finding is significant because it shows that the negative effects of AELEs may be reversible, thus preventing the transfer of the epigenetically altered genes associated with negative mental health outcomes across generations (National Scientific Council on the Developing Child 2010). Additionally, toxic stress can be reduced to tolerable stress or positive stress through protective factors. Particularly effective methods to reduce stress include having a supportive adult in the child's environment and safe, stable, and nurturing relationships (Centers for Disease Control and Prevention 2013c). Positive relationships can reduce toxic stress caused by AELEs, thus reducing the risk for long-term poor mental health and mental disorders.

Risk Factors for Adverse Early Life Experiences in the Clinical Setting

Case Example: A Multigenerational Approach to Adverse Early Life Experiences

Susan Williams is an 18-year-old high school senior, recently referred by a physician in a local obstetrics/gynecology clinic to Dr. Myra Johnson, a consulting psychiatrist, for evaluation of symptoms of fatigue, difficulty sleeping, loss of appetite, difficulty concentrating, and poor school attendance. Ms. Williams explains that she has not been feeling well for the past few months. Two months ago she found out that she is pregnant, and she is now 4 months along. This pregnancy was unplanned, but she and her boyfriend of 2 years, who is also a student, are looking forward to having the baby. Ms. Williams is living with her mother, who is angry about the pregnancy and is worried about how her daughter will balance finishing school and taking care of the baby. Her mother is currently working two jobs to make ends meet but still struggles financially.

Ms. Williams has no previous history of depressive symptoms and has never made a suicide attempt, although she did think of taking an overdose of pills on several occasions after arguments with her mother. She has no history of manic or hypomanic symptoms and no evidence of a thought disorder. She denies smoking or taking drugs, and although she admits to occasionally drinking with her friends, she says that she never has more than two drinks at a time. Ms. Williams states that she has lost about 5 pounds during her pregnancy, even though she has not had morning sickness. Until 2 months ago, she had been able to manage her schoolwork while working at a part-time job after school. Since becoming pregnant, she has had difficulty completing her schoolwork and several weeks ago quit her part-time job. She has not made any plans for what she would like to do when she finishes school.

The family history reveals that Ms. Williams's father, who had alcohol use disorder and cocaine use disorder, lived with her and her mother until about 10 years ago, when her parents separated. Her father would get into physical fights with her mother and insulted and criticized both Ms. Williams and her mother. Ms. Williams remembers that her father would occasionally hit her when she was young, but she does not remember ever requiring medical care for this abuse. In addition, one of her uncles touched her inappropriately; she told her mother, who banned him from visiting the house. Ms. Williams cannot confirm a history of depression in her mother, although her mother told her that she cried a lot for a few months after delivery (which Ms. Williams has always assumed to be evidence that her mother had not wanted her).

Assessing Adverse Early Life Experiences in the Clinical Setting

Dr. Johnson screened Ms. Williams for the presence of AELEs, which could be risk factors for the development of depression. Her history reveals that Ms. Williams experienced the following AELEs: viewing interpersonal violence between her parents, a household member with substance use disorders, experiencing emotional and physical abuse from her father and sexual abuse from an uncle, her mother's possible history of postpartum depression, and living without both of her biological parents since age 8.

Ms. Williams's symptoms of depression are complicated by her history of multiple AELEs, which puts her at increased risk for depressive disorders, anxiety disorders, suicide attempts, and substance use disorders. Additionally, she may have a genetic vulnerability to depression because of her mother's history of possible postpartum depression.

How Clinicians Can Address Adverse Early Life Experiences and Related Risk Factors

Screening Ms. Williams for a history of AELEs assists Dr. Johnson in developing a clinical care plan. Dr. Johnson plans to follow up with Ms. Williams to consider psychotherapy and possibly a medication for her depressive symptoms. Dr. Johnson will also monitor possible substance use and consider preventive interventions if necessary, ensure appropriate prenatal care, follow up with Ms. Williams in the postpartum period to address possible recurrent depression, and observe her relationship with her baby. An important step will be for Dr. Johnson to meet individuals in Ms. Williams's household or those involved in her social support system, namely, her mother and boyfriend. In doing so, Dr. Johnson will assess their availability to support Ms. Williams during her pregnancy and possible needs for individual or family interventions.

Ms. Williams's status as a single, teenage, first-time mother, as well as her history of emotional, physical, and sexual abuse (and witnessing physical abuse of her mother), places her at risk for neglect or abuse of her own child and at risk for being a victim of intimate partner violence in the future. Therefore, collaborating with other professionals, such as nurses or social workers, to provide additional services is recommended. For example, nurse-practitioners in the Nurse-Family Partnership program (Olds et al. 1997) provide regular home visits during pregnancy through 2 years postpartum. This evidence-based program reduces child maltreatment in at-risk mothers and assists mothers with managing school and/or return to work (Olds et al. 1997). Alternatively, eventual referral to a nurse or other clinician for parental skills training or to a social worker for financial assistance might also be indicated. Involving Ms. Williams's mother and boyfriend, treating Ms. Williams, and addressing Ms. Williams's eventual parenting skills—in other words, instituting a multigenerational approach—will assist both Ms. Williams and her child, thus preventing mental health problems from passing from one generation to the next.

Policy Approaches to Adverse Early Life Experiences as Social Determinants of Mental Health

In view of the widespread prevalence of AELEs such as childhood abuse and bullying, which are associated with further physical and mental health problems that are very costly to society as a whole, committing significant resources to reduce these social determinants of poor health is an urgent public health and national priority. Beyond the office, clinicians can have a broad impact on at-risk children and adolescents by advancing programs and policies at local, state, and federal levels and within education, health care, and legal systems. These efforts should emphasize the importance of early relationships that are safe, stable, and nurturing, with the overall strategy of strengthening families and communities.

Local and State Programs and Policies Addressing Adverse Early Life Experiences

Within one's local community, mental health professionals can provide information about the prevalence and impact of AELEs to local organizations such as parent-teacher associations and faith-based organizations and to child care and preschool professionals. These clinicians can encourage the expansion of programs and policies that are already in place or educate the community about interventions that need to be adopted. Within their professional organizations, mental health professionals can work on guidelines that promote AELE prevention. For example, in 2012, the American Academy of Pediatrics published "Early Childhood Adversity, Toxic Stress, and the Role of the Pediatrician: Translating Developmental Science into Lifelong Health," which recommended policy for incorporating preventive interventions for AELEs into clinical practice (Garner et al. 2012). Recognizing new advances in understanding the effects of early toxic stress on children, pediatricians can expand their roles to embrace wider activities to intervene on behalf of children and families at risk. Mental health professionals can do the same. Recommendations involve recognizing an *ecobiodevelopmental framework* (Garner et al. 2012; Shonkoff et al. 2012), which incorporates prevention and mental health promotion practices, as well as translating recent advances in neuroscience, genomics, molecular biology, and social sciences into tools that can be used in everyday practice. The Pediatric Medical Home model uses a developmental framework that recognizes how early experiences influence the health trajectory of the child into adulthood. Recommendations for practice in the Pediatric Medical Home model include preventive practices, screening at-risk children and families, collaborating with the community, and becoming advocates outside the clinical setting. Pediatricians have the potential to become more active leaders in educating the public and professionals about the consequences of toxic stress, the importance of treating children exposed to adversity, and learning more about effective interventions to prevent AELEs (Garner et al. 2012; Shonkoff et al. 2012). If they follow this approach, psychiatrists and other mental health professionals can also adapt these recommendations to everyday practice.

Additionally, mental health professionals can provide information to the media to educate the public about risk factors and preventive approaches after tragic occurrences, such as a suicide following bullying. They can also work with local advocacy organizations, state departments of education, legislators, and other stakeholders to recommend evidence-based programs to prevent AELEs. For example, in 2009, following news reports that an 11-year-old victim of bullying hanged himself, Georgia legislators passed a law requiring expansion of antibullying programs in Georgia's schools (Thomas-Whitfield 2011). Many states have adopted similar antibullying legislation in response to tragic events. Moreover, national advocacy organizations working through their local branches provide resources to promote child and family wellness and to prevent AELEs. Mental health professionals can act as consultants or participate on the advisory boards of these organizations.

State offices of child welfare/child protective services (CPS), public health, education, and juvenile justice all provide services to protect children's safety. CPS is charged with investigating reported cases of child abuse to determine if allegations of abuse are substantiated. Although CPS offices provide a range of family support and preventive interventions for families with confirmed cases of child maltreatment, recently, they have begun to refer families with unsubstantiated cases to community organizations offering similar services. Thus, instead of closing cases where suspected child abuse was not confirmed, providers may prescribe services to address family problems and prevent possible maltreatment for families about which they nevertheless remain concerned (Waldfogel 2009).

For the past 15 years, state departments of education have taken a more active role in providing safety to students through antibullying programs. Since 1999, legislation requiring school districts to implement policies addressing bullying has been passed in 49 states (Bully Police USA 2013). The laws are not uniform across all states, but much of the legislation defines bullying, recommends antibullying policies, or mandates antibullying programs in schools. The majority of states recognize cyberbullying as a threat as well. Although authority over bullying has traditionally been handled by school personnel, a recent trend toward handling more serious forms of bullying through the criminal justice system has arisen. Several states require that bullying incidents be reported to the state's department of education, many laws require that schools provide counseling and support services, and 16 states presently require that schools or districts provide staff training and professional development about bullying. Laws in most states require or encourage some type of bullying education or prevention program for students (Stuart-Cassel et al. 2011).

Federal Programs and National Initiatives Addressing Adverse Early Life Experiences

To protect and provide for the safety of maltreated children, the federal government passed the Child Abuse Prevention and Treatment Act (CAPTA) in 1974 (Child Welfare Information Gateway 2013b). This groundbreaking legislation and subsequent amendments provide federal funding to states in support of prevention, assessment, investigation, prosecution, and treatment activities as well as grants to public agencies and nonprofit organizations for demonstration projects and programs (Child Welfare Information Gateway 2013b). Although the primary responsibility for provision of child welfare services rests with state governments, the federal government supports states through funding and regulations for the care and reporting of maltreated children. As of 2012, statutes in 18 states require any person who suspects child abuse to submit a report to CPS, whereas other states legislate reporting by only certain professionals (Child Welfare Information Gateway 2013b). Although child welfare systems vary by state, their services include receiving and investigating reports of abuse and neglect, services to families to assist in protection and care of their children, arranging for children to live with relatives or foster families when the children are not safe at home, and planning for eventual permanent living arrangements through reunification with the family, adoption, or placement of individuals who age out of foster care (Child Welfare Information Gateway 2013b).

Although the responsibility for funding the implementation of child and family legislation rests within state and federal governments, other federal agencies, such as the CDC and the Substance Abuse and Mental Health Services Administration, administer additional research on and program grants for services related to interpersonal violence, child abuse prevention, and high-quality early education. The Division of Violence Prevention within CDC's National Center for Injury Prevention and Control is committed to the prevention of violence through surveillance, research and development, and capacity building (Centers for Disease Control and Prevention 2013d). Given the widespread prevalence of child maltreatment accompanied by serious negative long-term physical and mental health outcomes, the CDC sees child maltreatment as a significant threat to children's healthy development. In addition to collecting data about the prevalence of ACEs and risks for ACEs, the agency also tracks deaths of children due to maltreatment through the National Violent Death Reporting System (Centers for Disease Control and Prevention 2013d). These data are very helpful to practitioners, researchers, legislators, and the public in tracking the benefits of preventive interventions. Since the original ACE Study was published in 1998 (Felitti et al. 1998), many CDC researchers have collaborated on studying and reporting on the prevalence and clustering of ACEs and their long-term health consequences.

Bringing together research findings both from within the CDC and from around the country, researchers have developed a strategy for preventing child maltreatment through the promotion of *safe, stable, and nurturing relationships* between children and caregivers (Centers for Disease Control and Prevention 2013d). *Safety* of a child requires freedom from physical and emotional harm, *stability* refers to the need for children to be in a consistent and predictable environment associated with regular routines, and *nurturing* involves the ability of a caregiver to be sensitive and responsive to the child's needs (Centers for Disease Control and Prevention 2013d). Although these three characteristics are implemented in some prevention and promotion interventions, only a limited number of studies have operationalized these characteristics in detail to further document how they protect children, and few studies systematically promote them in a way that can be implemented broadly. To this end, as of 2013, the CDC is funding a multiyear study to be coordinated by five state health departments. The key focus will be addressing the social determinants of child maltreatment and safe, stable, and nurturing relationships, expanding beyond individual and family influences to community and societal factors as well (Centers for Disease Control and Prevention 2013c, 2013d).

A well-documented and long lasting prevention and promotion program providing high-quality early education to low-income families is the High/Scope Perry Preschool curriculum, which has been embedded into the national Head Start program. In 27- and 40-year follow-ups, participants in the High/Scope Perry Preschool program had significantly higher levels of school completion, greater monthly earnings, higher home ownership rates, lower rates of receiving welfare, and fewer arrests and incarcerations than the control group (Schweinhart and Weikart 1993; Schweinhart et al. 2005). The High/Scope Perry Preschool program curriculum and similar ones have been adopted in many Head Start programs, given the evidence for reducing negative behavioral outcomes through high-quality early education, parental support and parental skills training, and positive relationships.

Promoting Safe, Stable, and Nurturing Environments: A Role for Everyone

Everyone has a role in preventing AELEs and promoting safe, stable, and nurturing social environments. Given the widespread prevalence of AELEs, their considerable impact on children's lifelong physical and mental health, and their effects on the well-being of society as a whole, the prevention of AELEs is a high public health priority. In the clinical setting, mental health professionals can institute primary, secondary, or tertiary prevention, such as targeting at-risk children or families for preventive interventions, screening for depression in pregnant and postpartum women, or treating parents with substance use disorders. In addition, collaborations with the health, education, legislative, and judicial sectors, as well as with public and private organizations, will strengthen programs and policies to support healthy families and relationships. Furthermore, working as an advocate in one's professional organizations or in one's community can help educate people about the widespread prevalence of AELEs and promote recognition of the impact of related social determinants, such as poverty, income inequality, and racial discrimination. The confluence of all of these strategies will help not only children at risk but also their families, society, and future generations.

Key Points

- Adverse early life experiences are characterized by threatening and harmful relationships within homes and other caretaking environments. They are widespread and are social determinants of risky behaviors, poor mental health, and mental disorders.

- Research indicates that chronic child maltreatment and family dysfunction can lead to toxic stress (which can alter gene expression and brain development) and are risk factors for negative mental health outcomes.

- Routine evaluations and screening can identify risk factors for adverse early life experiences (e.g., the presence of family dysfunction, interpersonal violence, and perinatal depression). With a prevention-minded clinical approach, appropriate individual, family, and community interventions can be implemented.

- Community, state, and federal initiatives can reduce adverse early life experiences through programs (e.g., nurse home visits and school antibullying programs) and policies (e.g., mandated reporting of child abuse and providing services to at-risk families).

- Positive and consistent early life experiences, in which the young person has safe, stable, and nurturing relationships in his or her social environment, promote both physical and mental health throughout life. Individuals, communities, and institutions all have a responsibility to create safe, stable, and nurturing environments for growing children to promote their development into healthy and productive adults.

References

Agnafors S, Sydsjö G, Dekeyser L, et al: Symptoms of depression postpartum and 12 years later-associations to child mental health at 12 years of age. Matern Child Health J 17(3):405–414, 2013 22466717

Allen NB, Lewinsohn PM, Seeley JR: Prenatal and perinatal influences on risk for psychopathology in childhood and adolescence. Dev Psychopathol 10(3):513–529, 1998 9741680

Anda RF, Whitfield CL, Felitti VJ, et al: Adverse childhood experiences, alcoholic parents, and later risk of alcoholism and depression. Psychiatr Serv 53(8):1001–1009, 2002 12161676

Anda RF, Brown DW, Dube SR, et al: Adverse childhood experiences and chronic obstructive pulmonary disease in adults. Am J Prev Med 34(5):396–403, 2008 18407006

Arseneault L, Walsh E, Trzesniewski K, et al: Bullying victimization uniquely contributes to adjustment problems in young children: a nationally representative cohort study. Pediatrics 118(1):130–138, 2006 16818558

Borowsky IW, Taliaferro LA, McMorris BJ: Suicidal thinking and behavior among youth involved in verbal and social bullying: risk and protective factors. J Adolesc Health 53(1)(suppl):S4–S12, 2013 23790200

Brown DW, Anda RF, Tiemeier H, et al: Adverse childhood experiences and the risk of premature mortality. Am J Prev Med 37(5):389–396, 2009 19840693

Brunstein Klomek A, Sourander A, Gould M: The association of suicide and bullying in childhood to young adulthood: a review of cross-sectional and longitudinal research findings. Can J Psychiatry 55(5):282–288, 2010 20482954

Bully Police USA: Bully Police, May 2013. Available at: http://www.bullypolice.org. Accessed November 2, 2013.

Bynum L, Griffin T, Ridings DL, et al: Adverse childhood experiences reported by adults—five states, 2009. MMWR 59(49):1609–1613, 2010

Centers for Disease Control and Prevention: Understanding bullying. Atlanta, GA, Centers for Disease Control and Prevention, August 21, 2012. Available at: http://www.cdc.gov/violenceprevention/pub/understanding_bullying.html. Accessed October 20, 2013

Centers for Disease Control and Prevention: Adverse Childhood Experiences (ACE) Study Pyramid. Atlanta, GA, Centers for Disease Control and Prevention, 2013a. Available at: http://www.cdc.gov/ace/pyramid.htm. Accessed June 24, 2013.

Centers for Disease Control and Prevention: Adverse Childhood Experiences Study: major findings by publication year. Atlanta, GA, Centers for Disease Control and Prevention, January 18, 2013b. Available at: http://www.cdc.gov/ace/year.htm. Accessed February 17, 2014.

Centers for Disease Control and Prevention: Essentials for childhood: steps to create safe, stable, and nurturing relationships. Atlanta, GA, Centers for Disease Control and Prevention, 2013c. Available at: http://www.cdc.gov/violenceprevention/pdf/efc-01-03-2013-a.pdf. Accessed July 10, 2013.

Centers for Disease Control and Prevention: Promoting safe, stable, and nurturing relationships: A strategic direction for child maltreatment and prevention. Atlanta, GA, Centers for Disease Control and Prevention, 2013d.
Available at: http://www.cdc.gov/ViolencePrevention/pdf/CM_Strategic_
Direction--OnePager-a.pdf. Accessed November 5, 2013.

Child Welfare Information Gateway: Foster Care Statistics 2011. Washington, DC,
U.S. Department of Health and Human Services, Children's Bureau, 2013a.
Available at: http://www.childwelfare.gov/pubs/factsheets/foster.pdf.
Accessed July 23, 2013.

Child Welfare Information Gateway: How the Child Welfare System Works.
Washington, DC, U.S. Department of Health and Human Services, Children's Bureau, 2013b

Copper RL, Goldenberg RL, Das A, et al: The preterm prediction study: maternal stress is associated with spontaneous preterm birth at less than thirty-
five weeks' gestation. Am J Obstet Gynecol 175(5):1286–1292, 1996 8942502

Corwin DL: The Adverse Childhood Experiences Study: Background, Findings,
and Paradigm Shift. Shakopee, MN, Academy on Violence and Abuse, 2012

DiPietro JA: The role of prenatal maternal stress in child development. Curr Dir
Psychol Sci 13:71–74, 2004

Dong M, Giles WH, Felitti VJ, et al: Insights into causal pathways for ischemic
heart disease: adverse childhood experiences study. Circulation 110(13):1761–
1766, 2004 15381652

Draper B, Pfaff JJ, Pirkis J, et al: Long-term effects of childhood abuse on the
quality of life and health of older people: results from the Depression and
Early Prevention of Suicide in General Practice Project. J Am Geriatr Soc
56(2):262–271, 2008 18031482

Dube SR, Anda RF, Felitti VJ, et al: Childhood abuse, household dysfunction,
and the risk of attempted suicide throughout the life span: findings from the
Adverse Childhood Experiences Study. JAMA 286(24):3089–3096, 2001
11754674

Dube SR, Felitti VJ, Dong M, et al: Childhood abuse, neglect, and household
dysfunction and the risk of illicit drug use: the adverse childhood experiences study. Pediatrics 111(3):564–572, 2003 12612237

Dube SR, Fairweather D, Pearson WS, et al: Cumulative childhood stress and
autoimmune diseases in adults. Psychosom Med 71(2):243–250, 2009
19188532

Felitti VJ, Anda RF: The relationship of adverse childhood experiences to adult
medical disease, psychiatric disorders and sexual behavior: implications for
healthcare, in The Impact of Early Life Trauma on Health and Disease: The
Hidden Epidemic. Edited by Lanius RA, Vermetten E, Pain C. Cambridge,
UK, Cambridge University Press, 2010, pp 77–87

Felitti VJ, Anda RF, Nordenberg D, et al: Relationship of childhood abuse and
household dysfunction to many of the leading causes of death in adults. The
Adverse Childhood Experiences (ACE) Study. Am J Prev Med 14(4):245–
258, 1998 9635069

Finkelhor D, Turner H, Ormrod R, et al: Children's Exposure to Violence: A
Comprehensive National Survey. Juvenile Justice Bulletin. Rockville, MD,
U.S. Department of Justice, 2009

Gale CR, O'Callaghan FJ, Bredow M, et al: The influence of head growth in fetal life, infancy, and childhood on intelligence at the ages of 4 and 8 years. Pediatrics 118(4):1486–1492, 2006 17015539

Garner AS, Shonkoff JP, Seigel BS, et al: Early childhood adversity, toxic stress, and the role of the pediatrician: translating developmental science into lifelong health. Pediatrics 129(1):e224–e231, 2012 22201148

Gilbert LK: Behavioral Risk Factor Surveillance System Adverse Childhood Experiences Study: results from 10 U.S. states and the District of Columbia, 2010. Paper presented at the Epidemic Intelligence Service Conference, Atlanta, GA, April 2013

Hack M, Klein NK, Taylor HG: Long-term developmental outcomes of low birth weight infants. Future Child 5(1):176–196, 1995 7543353

Hatzenbuehler ML, Keyes KM: Inclusive anti-bullying policies and reduced risk of suicide attempts in lesbian and gay youth. J Adolesc Health 53(1)(suppl):S21–S26, 2013 23790196

Hay DF, Pawlby S, Sharp D, et al: Intellectual problems shown by 11-year-old children whose mothers had postnatal depression. J Child Psychol Psychiatry 42(7):871–889, 2001 11693583

Huizink AC, Mulder EJ, Buitelaar JK: Prenatal stress and risk for psychopathology: specific effects or induction of general susceptibility? Psychol Bull 130(1):115–142, 2004 14717652

LaPrairie JL, Heim CM, Nemeroff CB: The neuroendocrine effects of early life trauma, in The Impact of Early Life Trauma on Health and Disease: The Hidden Epidemic. Edited by Lanius RA, Vermetten E, Pain C. Cambridge, UK, Cambridge University Press, 2010, pp 157–165

Limber SP, Olweus D, Luxenberg H: Bullying in U.S. Schools: 2012 Status Report. Center City, MN, Hazelden Foundation, 2013

Lou HC, Hansen D, Nordentoft M, et al: Prenatal stressors of human life affect fetal brain development. Dev Med Child Neurol 36(9):826–832, 1994 7926332

Meijer A: Child psychiatric sequelae of maternal war stress. Acta Psychiatr Scand 72(6):505–511, 1985 2417452

Middlebrooks JS, Audage NC: The Effects of Childhood Stress on Health Across the Lifespan. Atlanta, GA, Centers for Disease Control and Prevention, 2008

Murray L, Sinclair D, Cooper P, et al: The socioemotional development of 5-year-old children of postnatally depressed mothers. J Child Psychol Psychiatry 40(8):1259–1271, 1999 10604404

Naicker K, Wickham M, Colman I: Timing of first exposure to maternal depression and adolescent emotional disorder in a national Canadian cohort. PLoS ONE 7(3):e33422, 2012 DOI: 10.1371/journal.pone.0033422 22461893

National Center on Family Homelessness: America's Youngest Outcasts 2010: State Report Card on Child Homelessness, 2011. Available at: http://www.homelesschildrenamerica.org/media/AYO%202010%20Fact%20Sheet_121211.pdf. Accessed July 22, 2013

National Scientific Council on the Developing Child: Excessive Stress Disrupts the Architecture of the Developing Brain, Working Paper No 3. Cambridge, MA, Harvard University, Center on the Developing Child, 2005

National Scientific Council on the Developing Child: Early Experiences Can Alter Gene Expression and Affect Long-Term Development: Working Paper No 10. Cambridge, MA, Harvard University, Center on the Developing Child, 2010

Norman RE, Byambaa M, De R, et al: The long-term health consequences of child physical abuse, emotional abuse, and neglect: a systematic review and meta-analysis. PLoS Med 9(11):e1001349, 2012 DOI: 10.1371/journal.pmed.1001349 23209385

O'Hara MW, Swain AM: Rates and risk of postpartum depression—a meta-analysis. Int Rev Psychiatry 8:37–54, 1996

Olds DL, Eckenrode J, Henderson CR Jr, et al: Long-term effects of home visitation on maternal life course and child abuse and neglect. Fifteen-year follow-up of a randomized trial. JAMA 278(8):637–643, 1997 9272895

Olweus D: Bullying at school: basic facts and effects of a school based intervention program. J Child Psychol Psychiatry 35(7):1171–1190, 1994 7806605

Philipps LH, O'Hara MW: Prospective study of postpartum depression: 4 1/2-year follow-up of women and children. J Abnorm Psychol 100(2):151–155, 1991 2040765

Rich-Edwards JW, Spiegelman D, Lividoti Hibert EN, et al: Abuse in childhood and adolescence as a predictor of type 2 diabetes in adult women. Am J Prev Med 39(6):529–536, 2010 21084073

Schweinhart LJ, Weikart DP: Success by empowerment: The High/Scope Perry Preschool study through age 27. Young Child 49:54–58, 1993

Schweinhart LJ, Montie J, Xiang Z, et al: The High/Scope Perry Preschool Study Through Age 40: Summary, Conclusions, and Frequently Asked Questions. Ypsilanti, MI, HighScope Educational Research Foundation, 2005

Shonkoff JP, Garner AS, Committee on Psychosocial Aspects of Child and Family Health, et al: The lifelong effects of early childhood adversity and toxic stress. Pediatrics 129(1):e232–e246, 2012 DOI: 10.1542/peds.2011–2663 22201156

Sourander A, Jensen P, Rönning JA, et al: What is the early adulthood outcome of boys who bully or are bullied in childhood? The Finnish "From a Boy to a Man" study. Pediatrics 120(2):397–404, 2007 17671067

Stuart-Cassel V, Bell A, Springer JF: Analysis of State Bullying Laws and Policies. Washington, DC, U.S. Department of Education, 2011. Available at: http://www2.ed.gov/rschstat/eval/bullying/state-bullying-laws/state-bullying-laws.pdf. Accessed November 13, 2013.

Thomas-Whitfield C: Jaheem Hererra's suicide inspired lawmakers to beef up Georgia's school bullying policies. Juvenile Justice Information Exchange, October 26, 2011. Available at: http://jjie.org/jaheem-herreras-suicide-inspired-lawmakers-beef-up-georgias-school-bullying-policies/40238/2/. Accessed November 13, 2013.

U.S. Department of Health and Human Services: Child Maltreatment. Washington, DC, U.S. Department of Health and Human Services, 2012. Available at: http://www.acf.hhs.gov/programs/cb/research-data-technology/statistics-research/child-maltreatment. Accessed November 13, 2013.

Waldfogel J: Prevention and the child protection system. Future of Children 19:195–210, 2009

Walker EA, Gelfand A, Katon WJ, et al: Adult health status of women with histories of childhood abuse and neglect. Am J Med 107(4):332–339, 1999 10527034

Whitfield CL, Anda RF, Dube SR: Violent childhood experiences and the risk of intimate partner violence in adults: assessment in a large health maintenance organization. J Interpers Violence 18:166–185, 2003

Whitfield CL, Dube SR, Felitti VJ, et al: Adverse childhood experiences and hallucinations. Child Abuse Negl 29(7):797–810, 2005 16051353

Widom CS, Czaja SJ, Bentley T, et al: A prospective investigation of physical health outcomes in abused and neglected children: new findings from a 30-year follow-up. Am J Public Health 102(6):1135–1144, 2012 22515854

4

Poor Education

Rebecca A. Powers, M.D., M.P.H.

*The school is the last expenditure upon which
America should be willing to economize.*

Franklin D. Roosevelt, 1882–1945

The environments in which people learn, at all ages, directly and indirectly affect their health and well-being. Better education portends better health. Individuals who are less educated are less able to secure jobs with optimal pay, which puts them at greater risk for poor health than those with higher socioeconomic status (SES). These associations are significant across the entire life span. For example, the higher one's education, the lower one's rates of chronic diseases such as osteoarthritis and hypertension, as well as certain cancers such as cervical cancer. The likelihood of having diverse illnesses—ranging from minor ones such as headaches or upper respiratory infections to major and serious ones such as coronary heart disease—is increased by poor education. Several pathways are involved in these undoubtedly complex associations (Matthews and Gallo 2011). In this chapter the focus is on the relations between poor education (at both the individual and community levels) and poor mental health outcomes, as well as steps that both clinicians and policy makers, and indeed everyone, can take to enhance education and thus promote health.

As social beings, we need to feel a sense of belonging and of being valued, appreciated, loved, and understood. That feeling begins in the home but is reinforced in the school setting, which is the most influential social setting during childhood and adolescence. Aside from the academic attainment that might be seen as the primary task of schooling, there are many other meaningful psychological and social skills learned in the school environment, including relationships, social support and coping abilities, cognitive capacity, social norms and values, the meaning of work, self-regulation and control, and frustration tolerance. If we do not adequately learn these valuable assets and skills, we are more prone to depression, anxiety, hostility, and feelings of hopelessness, helplessness, and worthlessness. These negative emotions can affect our ability to cope with stress and guard against preventable mental and physical illnesses. In addition, in school settings, screenings can be quickly performed, health information can be easily gathered, and preventive interventions can be effectively delivered.

As childhood education is required by the United States and most other societies, most children in the United States receive their education in public primary and secondary schools. However, the quality of education in the United States is below that of many other Western countries. In one report, the United States ranked seventeenth in education quality in the developed world, with Finland, South Korea, Hong Kong, Japan, and Singapore at the top (Economist Intelligence Unit 2014). Furthermore, students in many other countries are making academic gains at a much faster pace than those in the United States (Hanushek et al. 2012). Clearly, there is room for improvement in education in the United States. Such improvement will enhance health.

It is our duty to ensure that school settings are safe and health-promoting environments. Schools build human qualities, including those that promote health and reduce risk for disease, while providing the education that becomes a pathway for a high quality of life in adulthood. Good health is related to good education in several ways. With more schooling, people can earn more money, which leads to better overall opportunities, an ability to reside in safer neighborhoods, improved interpersonal relationships, better parenting, richer social networks, and improved quality of life. Furthermore, with greater education and better earnings, individuals have access to healthier food choices and higher-quality medical care and thus a greater opportunity to achieve physical and mental wellness. As a result, low education is one of many major social determinants of mental disorders (Patel 2007).

A natural lag exists between education and health outcomes. One usually experiences health consequences as an adult, after completing one's education (although an increasing trend of negative health consequences, such as obesity and depression, manifesting in children and adolescents has arisen); therefore, in terms of the direction of causality, poor education typically precedes poor health outcomes, and adult health probably does not affect one's level of educational attainment. By contrast, childhood illnesses and low birth weight can contribute to lower educational achievement (Case et al. 2002). Thus, ~~SES and educational attainment affect health, and in a reciprocal fashion, health~~ affects ~~educational attainment to some extent.~~

In recent years, many efforts have been made at the local, state, and federal levels to improve the quality of education in the United States, ranging from early childhood education to higher education. Although these programs and policies typically focus on enhancing education per se as the outcome or goal of interest, in this chapter we demonstrate how such efforts also indirectly improve health. Improving the quality of education will ultimately promote both physical health and mental health and will reduce the risk of physical and mental illnesses. As such, clinicians have a central role in the ongoing discourse about education reform at the local, state, and federal levels, and such involvement will undoubtedly improve the health of the nation in due course.

Although the focus of this chapter is poor education as a social determinant of mental health and related clinical and policy implications, many topics that are very important to any discussion of the interface between education and mental health are beyond the purview of this chapter. At least three such topics are noteworthy. First, bullying in the school setting is increasingly recognized as detrimental to immediate and long-term mental health outcomes. Bullying as an adverse early life experience (and thus a social determinant of mental health) is discussed in Chapter 3, "Adverse Early Life Experiences." Second, suicide in mid- dle and high school and college settings is a tragedy that is increasing in prevalence in the United States. Many programs are being developed to address this crucial problem, with a goal of preventing suicide and facilitating referral to services for students who are at risk for suicide. Third, although in this chapter the focus is on educational quality and equality with regard to students in general, some students can excel only when provided with special accommodations. Improving and expanding such accommodations, whether they are needed for learning, attentional, physical, or other limitations, are vital in conjunction with more general efforts to reduce the risks associated with poor education.

Poor Education as a Social Determinant of Health

Educational attainment affects health by enhancing brain development; conveying health literacy; encouraging the development of healthy behaviors; allowing children to develop a sense of control, achievement, and empowerment; and lending greater employment and income opportunities across the life span. Poor education is associated with diverse adverse health outcomes. For example, higher educational level, rather than personal income, may be protective against overweight and obesity in women. Being overweight or obese, in turn, affects many aspects of health and well-being. Therefore, it has been suggested that obesity prevention efforts should target those with socioeconomic disadvantage and those with poor education (Williams et al. 2013). Educational level is inversely associated with life stress as well as social isolation, both of which are linked to increased risk for myocardial infarction and cardiac death (Ruberman et al. 1984). Graduating from high school is associated with decreased risky health behaviors, reduced burden of illness, delays in the consequences of aging, increased life expectancy, and decreased disparities in health. Risky health behaviors such as smoking, being overweight, and having a sedentary lifestyle are related directly to having less schooling (Freudenberg and Ruglis 2007).

Poor education can impact health in many ways, one of which pertains to the recognition that disadvantaged environments expose individuals to greater stress. Allostasis and the degree of allostatic load are a conceptual model that might explain health disparities in those experiencing cumulative stress. Endocrine, metabolic, cardiovascular, and immune systems are all altered by chronic stress. Both less education and lower income predict higher allostatic load scores (McEwen and Seeman 1999), and individuals experiencing greater allostatic load have poorer physical health and cognitive functioning (Seeman et al. 2001). Cardiovascular disease, diabetes, asthma, cervical cancer, depression, disability, and mortality are all greater in those at the lowest levels of education and income (Adler and Rehkopf 2008).

Having more formal education is linked to lower death rates and later death. In a fascinating analysis by Galea and colleagues (2011), the numbers of deaths in the United States attributable to six social factors were estimated using data from a host of prior studies. Galea et al. (2011) found that in 2000, approximately 245,000 deaths were attributable to low education (defined as less than a high school education compared with a high school diploma equivalent or greater). With regard to the other social factors examined, 176,000 deaths were attributable to racial segregation, 162,000 to low social support, 133,000 to poverty, 119,000 to income inequality, and 39,000 to area-level poverty. The authors noted that these mortality estimates are comparable to deaths from the leading pathophysiological causes (e.g., the number of deaths attributable to low education was comparable to the number caused by acute myocardial infarction). Although these six factors are very much interrelated to one another, the shocking findings indicate a major need for policy action to address these social determinants of health, and improving educational attainment must be at the top of the list.

Poor Education as a Social Determinant of Mental Health

Several factors influence whether a child receives a poor or a high-quality education. Stressful events in the life of a child and his or her family contribute to anxiety, insecurity, low self-esteem, social isolation, and a sense of lack of control over school and home life, all of which impact education and have their own formidable effects on physical and mental health. Cognitive, emotional, and sensory inputs program the developing brain's responses to stressful conditions or life experiences both at home and at school. Adverse societal factors can lead to insecure emotional attachment and poor stimulation, which can set the stage for reduced readiness for school, low educational attainment, problem behaviors, and the risk of being socially disadvantaged in adulthood. Parental and peer group role modeling, especially in the school setting, affects health-related habits such as eating nutritious foods, exercising, not smoking, abstaining from drugs, managing time successfully, having healthful activities inside and outside of school, and using adaptive coping strategies. Children learn better if they are not on guard to protect themselves from the insecurities and threats in their neighborhoods, on the school grounds, or during transit to and from school each day. Families whose household members have less than a high school education report more stressful events than those headed by a high school or college graduate (Dohrenwend and Dohrenwend 1973).

One cannot discuss poor education without addressing poverty or low SES because an obvious strong link exists between poverty and low income and poor education. Although these two social determinants of health are difficult to separate, absolute and relative poverty are discussed in Chapter 6, "Economic Inequality, Poverty, and Neighborhood Deprivation." Like poverty and income inequality, social exclusion that results from racism, discrimination, and stigma prevents people from fully participating in education or training and thus from gaining access to further opportunities and social mobility. A child's life can be affected dramatically by these social influences in his or her family, influences that are usually completely outside of the child's control. Schools within low-SES communities often have high student-to-teacher ratios, provide poorer quality of instruction, and lack adequate academic resources, all of which influence cognitive, social, and language development (Perkins et al. 2013). Therefore, the school environment deserves special attention in any discussion of the social determinants of mental health. Education is also linked to other important variables such as social support, feeling that one is part of a social network, and social integration. Those with lower SES have lower levels of these psychological and social protective factors, which directly contribute to resilience against poor mental health and also lead to poorer education. Socialization and life experiences that influence psychological development—an important asset gained from school settings—affect ongoing mood, affect, cognition, and health behaviors (Adler et al. 1994).

Although any discussion of education as a social determinant of mental health undoubtedly focuses largely on children and adolescents, educational attainment also affects the health of adults and the elderly. The educational attainment of one's parents also appears to be associated with health outcomes. The 2003 National Comorbidity Survey Replication Study showed that both socioeconomic disadvantage and having a depressed mother during one's youth increased the risk for adulthood major depression and/or chronic pain. If the parents also had lower educational attainment, chronic pain increased in magnitude across adulthood compared with those with higher education. As such, social factors clearly help to explain some of the complexities in adulthood physical and mental health outcomes (Goosby 2013).

Parent-child interactions have an irrefutable effect on developing children at every socioeconomic level. Parents with greater education likely have greater ability to teach more effectively and support their children's learning. Educational status also impacts mental health through its associations with mental health literacy (i.e., the knowledge and beliefs about mental disorders that help in their recognition, management, and prevention) (Kaneko and Motohashi 2007).

Early Childhood

Early childhood is a crucial time in human development, and difficulties at home or school can affect mental and physical health in many ways. A high-quality prekindergarten experience can have diverse, long-term benefits in children's lives, as well as in the lives of their parents and their future children (Schulman 2005). Studies of several early childhood interventions, including the High/Scope Perry Preschool Program, the Abecedarian Project, Chicago Child-Parent Centers, and Parent-Child Development Centers, document that children who participate in a high-quality early childhood education experience gains beyond the commonly emphasized educational benefits.

The High/Scope Perry Preschool Study was a scientific experiment that identified both the short- and long-term effects of a high-quality preschool education program for young children living in poverty. Designed to help preschool children avoid later school failure and related problems, it was ultimately found to accomplish much more. The study involved a 2-year preschool education program for 3- and 4-year-olds living in low-income families. Teachers each served five or six children, and they had bachelor's degrees, certification in education, and regular training and support. The High/Scope educational model was used in daily 2-hour classes with weekly family visits. Teachers promoted children's self-initiated learning activities, provided both small-group and large-group activities, and focused on key experiences in child development.

Over the years, the High/Scope study has produced eight monographs with many types of results. The findings on this program's effects on participants through age 40 span the domains of education, economic performance, crime prevention, family relationships, and health. Some of the key findings for participants at age 40 years are summarized in Table 4–1. The major conclusion of the study is that high-quality preschool programs for young children living in poverty contribute to their intellectual and social development in childhood and school success, economic performance, and reduced crime in adulthood. The initial investment in the program is even more worthwhile than originally estimated (Schweinhart et al. 2005).

Much has also been learned about the prominent health and social benefits of high-quality early childhood education from Head Start, a federal program implemented locally that provides preschoolers with education and health services. This program is the foremost U.S. federally funded provider of educational services to young children living in poverty. Since 1965, more than 30 million children have participated in this comprehensive child development program. Head Start not only mandates educational services but also provides social, health, and nutritional services to children and their low-income parents. When Early Head Start was established in 1994, the program was expanded to serve even younger children (from birth to age 3) and their families. Head Start uses one of three types of systems, including the High/Scope Perry Preschool Program, which has the most established outcomes overall.

TABLE 4–1.   Major findings from the High/Scope Perry Preschool
                  Study

	Received the High/Scope Perry Preschool intervention	Did not receive the High/Scope Perry Preschool intervention
Graduated from high school	77%	60%
Earned ≥$20,000 at age 40	60%	40%
Arrested ≥5 times by age 40	36%	55%
IQ ≥90 at age 5	67%	28%

Source.   Schweinhart et al. 2005

Controversy exists over whether Head Start produces lasting benefits. Studies show increased intelligence quotient (IQ), but relative increases appear to fade over time. Many other studies find decreases in
grade retention and special education placements. Early Head Start demonstrated modest improvements in children's development and parents'
beliefs and behaviors. However, Head Start's budget remains insufficient
to serve all eligible children or deliver uniformly high-quality services to
those enrolled (Gormley et al. 2010).

Although school-based programs are clearly important, children obviously also learn at home. The *home literacy environment* can influence
a child's language development; for example, it has effects on kindergarten literacy skills, as well as effects into adulthood. In addition to
cognitive skills, the early home literacy environment affects kindergar-
teners' vocabulary and conceptual knowledge, which helps them with
printed word recognition and thus reading ability. Parental SES and parental reading to children are positive influences on the home literacy
environment. Maternal depression has negative impacts on the home
literacy environment, whereas maternal education positively affects it
(Perkins et al. 2013). One example of a program designed to enhance the
home literacy environment is Reach Out and Read, which targets parents of children from birth to 3 years by giving them books at pediatric
visits and encouraging them to read to their children.

Kindergarten Through High School

Multiple contexts, including family characteristics (e.g., the home literacy environment and parental involvement in school) and school and neighborhood conditions, combine to drive young children's reading achievement and partly account for the robust association between SES and reading outcomes (Aikens and Barbarin 2008). Living in a high-SES neighborhood is positively associated with children's IQ and educational attainment among older adolescents. The presence in the community of learning activities and venues, such as literacy programs, libraries, family resource centers, and museums, may influence children's development, especially in terms of school readiness and achievement outcomes. School sports programs, art and theater programs, community centers, and youth groups promote children's physical, social, and emotional well-being.

Beneficial school characteristics have been identified with regard to promoting positive social and emotional health outcomes. Small class size provides positive cognitive and academic outcomes (Muennig and Woolf 2007). Well-trained teachers with collegial support and good wages are key, and child-focused communication between home and school needs to be continued throughout the time the child is in school (Frede 1995). Specific curricula for promoting a positive school environment show clear impacts on students' mental health. Children in prekindergarten and kindergarten who are introduced to methods and content of material that are similar to what they will experience in elementary school benefit over those without the same curricular continuity.

One's level of education has prominent effects on health and social outcomes. Perhaps most important, dropping out of school before high school graduation has consistently been shown to be detrimental. In the United States, from 1975 through 2000, the percentage of young adults who graduated from high school increased from 63% to 84%. Unfortunately, however, the number of high school dropouts increased among low-income and black and Latino students. The rate at which those between ninth and tenth grade leave school tripled. Whites, women, and U.S.-born residents have higher graduation rates than their respective counterparts. The largest cities in the United States have the lowest graduation rates, and those with low-average incomes and a high proportion of black and Latino students fare the most poorly (Freudenberg and Ruglis 2007). Contributing factors are complex, but school dropout can be related to substance use and teenage pregnancy, as well as psychological, emotional, and behavioral problems. Families with medical, financial, or psychological needs can also give rise to youth dropping out of school to be of assistance at home.

Some states have mandated an increase in the dropout age. This change keeps students in school longer and thus increases their educational attainment. As a result, their earnings in adulthood increase, as well as their children's future educational attainment expectations. Dropping out of high school affects future educational and employment trajectories and is relevant to diverse health outcomes. The General Educational Development (GED) certificate or credential—often referred to as the General Equivalency Diploma—is available as an equivalent to a high school diploma for students who fail to complete high school. The health benefit associated with earning a GED is less than that of having a high school diploma, but it is nonetheless better than dropping out and not attaining a GED (Cohen and Syme 2013).

College Years

College is achieved more assuredly with a high school diploma, and completing college offers more health and mental health advantage than high school alone. College completion is associated with higher social and economic status and increased quality-adjusted life expectancy (Cohen and Syme 2013). Given that greater education overall is linked to better physical and mental health, it can be assumed that college graduation is linked to better mental health overall, although limited data are available. Note that mental health is predictive of college success, and the mental health needs of college students are increasingly being recognized (Hyun et al. 2006; Kitzrow 2003).

Poor Education as a Social Determinant of Mental Health: Clinical Considerations

Case Example: First Year in Middle School

Johnny Singer is a 13-year-old boy who is brought to the county community mental health center by his mother, Clara Singer, for signs and symptoms consistent with depression. Ms. Singer reports that since starting middle school several months ago, Johnny has had a hard time falling asleep and no longer feels like playing basketball with his friends. She also notices that he looks sad most of the time and has been getting bad grades because he has difficulty concentrating in class and does not feel like doing his homework. Also, he has lost some weight during the past few months and does not see himself as very smart or popular at school. Ms. Singer is a single parent and works full time as a waitress in a local diner. Johnny's father left Ms. Singer before Johnny was born.

The psychiatrist, Dr. Vera Hsu, is familiar with Johnny's middle school; it is known to receive insufficient funding and to have major capital needs, and it is located in a neighborhood with substantial crime and high rates of unemployment. Johnny tells Dr. Hsu that he wants to do well in school, but "I'm not very smart and I just can't focus." As Dr. Hsu talks further to Johnny, he openly describes his situation as follows:

"I'm always worried about my mom at the diner. There have been some bad fights there. And at home, I've heard gunshots at night and now I can't sleep. I'm the man of the house, and my mom and little sister can't do anything if somebody robs us." When asked about school, he says, "The teachers don't care about me, and one of them can't even remember my name. My mom tells me to do my homework, but she can't really help me with it. I really don't know how to do my homework most of the time, so I usually just skip it. I can't play basketball anymore after school, which is the only thing I liked doing before." Johnny also describes to Dr. Hsu that he would feel more motivated to do his homework if he could play basketball, but his mother won't let him walk to the court down the street because it is not lit well and she is concerned for his safety. Johnny tells Dr. Hsu that his school is "the worst" and that he doesn't really think about his future that much.

Johnny is clearly struggling in his neighborhood, at his middle school, and at home. His depressive symptoms seem to be intimately connected with his school situation. Already at risk in many ways, his poor education (and risk of academic failure and school dropout) places him at risk for additional social determinants of poor health (e.g., reduced employability in the future and lower likelihood of adequate income) and long-term poor mental and physical health. In addition to treating his depressive syndrome, Dr. Hsu has an opportunity to intervene in a way that might set him on a better path for educational attainment and success. On the basis of the diagnosis of depression, Dr. Hsu can assist with accommodations that could help Johnny resume playing basketball safely and receive tutoring through the school system.

Assessing Poor Education as a Risk Factor in the Clinical Setting

Clinicians can assess educational status and school activities with each new evaluation and, especially for youth and young adults, frequently during follow-up. Obtaining a chronological history of education is paramount, and questions can be broken down into elementary, middle, and high school blocks of time. For each of those blocks, questions for parents should include the school name, ages of attendance, type of school, experience, reports, testing, relationships with teachers, and relationships with other students. It is important to inquire about all aspects of educational success and psychosocial development that occur during the school years, including mastery and autonomy, object relations, obedience, performance, ability to work independently, how difficulty with homework is handled, extracurricular activities, sexual identity, and aspirations at each grade level. Specific symptoms at each grade level can be assessed, and any concerns of teachers or parents should be elicited. Additionally, the clinician can develop an understanding of the patient's individualized educational plans or instructional modifications if any exist. The clinician can also be aware of any school disciplinary actions, the nature of peer and family relationships, involvement in religious activities and hobbies, any legal issues, exposure to any past or ongoing adverse early life events, including bullying, and the patient's goals. Finally, for children and adolescents who appear to have attentional or learning difficulties that interfere with effective learning and academic achievement, it is crucial for the clinician 1) to get the appropriate neuropsychological evaluation, 2) to use results to obtain suitable accommodations for those difficulties in the school setting, and 3) to follow up to ensure that needed supports are available for the youth to excel in and complete school.

How Clinicians Can Address Poor Education

In clinical settings that embrace the recovery paradigm in which patients are empowered to acquire the tools necessary to achieve their own goals, young adults with psychiatric disabilities who have educational goals can be offered the psychosocial treatment called *supported education.* Deemed a promising practice by the U.S. Substance Abuse and Mental Health Services Administration, supported education is an established but inadequately disseminated psychosocial treatment that has an available implementation tool kit (Substance Abuse and Mental Health Services Administration 2012). It is a process for helping individuals with a diagnosis of a mental illness participate in an education program so they may receive the education and training they need to achieve their learning and recovery goals and become gainfully employed in the job or career of their choice (Substance Abuse and Mental Health Services Administration 2012). A number of studies indicate that supported education programs are associated with positive outcomes such as graduation (e.g., high school diploma or GED), development of improved interpersonal and work-related skills (e.g., social interactions in the workplace), a higher likelihood of employment, and positive self-esteem (Cook and Solomon 1993; Hoffman and Mastrianni 1993; Unger et al. 1991).

Beyond the walls of the clinic, health care providers can be involved in their local school district to promote policies around positive changes in the school environment. Clinicians, including psychiatrists and other mental health professionals, can help with education about suicide prevention strategies in schools, improving the healthfulness of school lunches, antibullying interventions, and other issues pertinent to promoting health in the school setting and reducing the risk of adverse social and mental health outcomes. Clinicians also can help boost community resources, such as libraries, family resource centers, literacy programs, museums, arts programs, and recreational facilities, that will support and enhance healthy youth development. Clinicians can provide educational materials on healthy youth development for distribution to patients and families in the offices of pediatricians and mental health professionals. Importantly, equal educational opportunities for all can be addressed in local school districts and communities.

Policy Considerations Pertaining to Poor Education

It has been noted that "formal education—from preschool to beyond college—is also one of the social determinants of health for which there are clear policy pathways for intervention" (Cohen and Syme 2013, p. 997). A fundamental goal in public health research and practice is to eliminate or at least significantly minimize mental health disparities in the United States. The causes of disparities are many and complex, but research has clearly demonstrated the links between poor education and health disparities in the United States. Improvement in education across society can bring about a reduction in mental health inequities. Although the United States no longer has formally segregated schools, many schools are located in neighborhoods characterized by little racial diversity, and further efforts to address informal segregation could improve educational quality for the socially disadvantaged.

Policies that promote education and educational equality are ultimately health policies. Promoting good health involves reducing educational failure and premature school dropout. Both the quantity and quality of education must be addressed. Administrative and institutional beliefs, the teachers themselves, classroom interactions, and the environment in which the institution is placed all need to be optimized. Small classroom size with low ratios of students to teachers and well-trained teachers with collegial support and good wages are key. Child-focused communication between home and school needs to be continued throughout the time the child is in school. Partnerships between school and family can be supported. Affordable, enticing, and healthier options for school lunches are also crucial for learning success. Health information can be gathered, and preventive interventions delivered, in the school setting. Thus, school-based clinics offer the opportunity for mental health promotion activities, screening for early detection of adverse mental health outcomes, and increasing access to mental health services.

In addition to local efforts, state and federal policy can have far-reaching impacts on education. In the United States, the federal role in education is limited, because the Tenth Amendment to the U.S. Constitution requires that most education policy be decided at the state and local levels. Nonetheless, a number of federal policy initiatives have been proposed and enacted to improve education. The most comprehensive in recent years is the controversial No Child Left Behind Act of 2001, a 670-page public law with diverse provisions, some of which are summarized in Table 4–2.

Also at the federal level, the American Recovery and Reinvestment Act of 2009—historic legislation designed to stimulate the economy, support job creation, and invest in critical sectors, including education—provided $4.35 billion for the Race to the Top Fund. This fund is a competitive grant program designed to encourage and reward states that are creating conditions for educational innovation and reform and attaining significant improvement in student achievement, graduation rates, and college and career preparation.

At the state and local levels, a multitude of policy and programmatic approaches can be pursued to improve the quality of education; two examples include the growth of charter schools and the use of voucher programs. Many urban leaders, such as mayors and school district superintendents, are initiating publicly supported charter schools that operate autonomously, which is thought to be a means of improving learning (Zimmer and Buddin 2006). Charter schools are founded on the thought that increasing choice and competition will foster innovation in education in terms of curricula, teaching methods, and teacher hiring and training practices. However, whether charter schools necessarily lead to better educational outcomes is unclear. A study in North Carolina indicated that students who transferred into charter schools made smaller gains than they would have if they had remained in tra-

TABLE 4-2. Key provisions of the No Child Left Behind Act of 2001

Increase accountability for states, school districts, and schools.
- For example, states should implement annual testing for all students in the third through eighth grades and annual statewide progress objectives ensuring that all groups of students reach proficiency in reading and mathematics within 12 years.
- Depending on results, school districts and schools may be subject to corrective actions or may be eligible for achievement awards.

Give greater choice for parents and students, particularly those attending low-performing schools, to help ensure that no child loses the opportunity for a quality education because he or she is trapped in a failing school.

Allow for more flexibility for states and local educational agencies in the use of federal education dollars, including funding received under four major state grant programs: Teacher Quality State Grants, Educational Technology, Innovative Programs, and Safe and Drug-Free Schools.

Create a stronger emphasis on reading, especially for the nation's youngest children.
- For example, the Reading First initiative significantly increased federal investment in scientifically based reading instruction programs in the early grades, and the Early Reading First program made competitive 6-year awards to local educational agencies to support early language, literacy, and prereading development of preschool-age children, particularly those from low-income families.

Mandate that states must allow students who attend a persistently dangerous school or who are victims of violent crime at school to transfer to a safe school.
- States also must report school safety statistics to the public on a school-by-school basis, and local educational agencies must use federal Safe and Drug-Free Schools and Communities funding to implement drug and violence prevention programs of demonstrated effectiveness.

ditional public schools, which might be partially explained by a higher student turnover rate in charter schools (Bifulco and Ladd 2006). An analysis from Florida suggested, however, that by their fifth year of operation, new charter schools were on par with average traditional public schools in math and produced higher reading achievement scores than their traditional public school counterparts (Sass 2006). Student achievement results show that charter schools are having mixed overall effects (and are generally not promoting student achievement for minority students) (Zimmer and Buddin 2006), and study results appear to vary by geographic region (Betts and Tang 2011). Therefore, additional research is needed on the effectiveness of charter schools (Miron and Nelson 2004), especially for minority groups across diverse areas. Publicly funded education voucher programs could allow parents to use public funds to enroll their child in a public or private school of their choosing (as a means of increasing choice and competition). Such programs are implemented much less frequently than charter schools, and research on their effectiveness in the United States is thus very limited.

Policy and Programs Pertaining to Early Childhood Education

Public policy can bring about changes at the preschool level and lead to significant influences on mental health. Findings from the High/Scope Perry Preschool Study and related studies have motivated policy makers to invest more in preschool programs. However, because lawmakers must often engage in political compromise, these programs have seldom been adequately disseminated and funded. The High/Scope Perry Preschool Study serves as a symbol of what government programs can and ought to strive to achieve. The High/Scope Perry Preschool, Abecedarian, and Chicago programs described in the section "Early Childhood" all confer significant benefits. Although they illuminate different aspects of the question of lasting effects of high-quality preschool education, they all reflect the same challenge of providing such programs that include low-income children so that these children can have a fair chance to achieve their potential and contribute meaningfully to their families and to society (Schweinhart et al. 2005). These gold standard programs have often been scaled back because of limited financial resources. Head Start programs also vary from state to state. Because high-quality Head Start programs have a more robust positive impact than those of lower quality, program fidelity must be supported with adequate resources.

Aside from local, state, and federal governments, the corporate sector could also have a role in ensuring equal and high-quality educational opportunities that ultimately promote health. Day care programs could be provided by more companies where parents are employed, and standards should exist for community programs. As indicated in the section "Early Childhood," the home literacy environment influences a child's language development; thus, programs such as Reach Out and Read should be offered for all demographic groups.

Policy and Programs Pertaining to Kindergarten Through High School

Primary and secondary schools exert a prominent influence on the health and development of children and adolescents, and the level of educational attainment, including high school graduation, is linked to diverse other social determinants of mental health. When needed, state-mandated policies to raise the dropout age should be supported to keep adolescents in school longer. GED tests need to be offered as an equivalency to a high school diploma for all students who drop out of school. The importance of a high school diploma always needs to be stressed as a critical public health objective. Policy makers and clinicians alike can learn from extensive educational research. Table 4–3 summarizes some of the many recommendations for improving student engagement in school and academic success (Freudenberg and Ruglis 2007).

Policy and Programs Pertaining to Higher Education

Higher education settings are another place to influence individuals' health and well-being. A degree or credential obtained, rather than just the years of education completed, is clearly beneficial in the long term. Policies that enable more high school graduates to go to college and successfully complete college will have a long-term impact on both individual and population health. Federal, state, and local governments need to continue to fund colleges, including local community colleges, so that they are all of high quality (e.g., with small class sizes and well-trained and talented professors). Because depression, problem drinking, and other behavioral disorders influence performance in school, screening for such problems on admission to colleges and universities, and periodically thereafter, could detect those at risk so that they can be provided with needed support and services.

TABLE 4-3. Summary of educational interventions for improving student engagement in school and academic success

Structural, institutional, and organizational changes
- Student involvement in school policies
- Reducing grade retention and suspension
- Parent and family training and involvement
- Violence prevention and conflict resolution programs

Changes to curriculum and instruction
- Extended class periods or increased instructional time
- Opportunities for "catch-up" courses and for out-of-school programs
- Tutoring and mentoring programs
- Interdisciplinary instruction

Changes to teacher support
- Highly qualified, certified, and well-prepared teachers
- Teachers teaching only in their field of certification
- Education programs to help teachers promote social justice
- Teacher training for effective instruction of and care for culturally and linguistically diverse learners

Source.   Freudenberg and Ruglis 2007

Improving Education: A Role for Everyone

Educational attainment and high-quality education are crucial for improving physical and mental health outcomes in the United States. Whereas local governments, the business community, and individual citizens might have little involvement in the development of medical interventions, they can all play a role in policy decisions and program development pertaining to improving education. Mental health professionals and other clinicians can advocate for improving educational quality in addition to screening and assisting children and families with resources for improving education. Clinicians can have a role in enhancing the home literacy environment for children in the preschool years. Then, with regard to kindergarten through high school and beyond, clinicians and all citizens can work to ensure that the school setting is an opportune site for interventions that overcome social class inequities, which, in turn, will reduce health inequities (Cohen and Syme 2013).

Educational policy and program proposals are frequently, if not continuously, being discussed at the local, state, and federal levels. Every citizen has a role in the discourse on diverse educational policies. Such policies range from implementation and funding of Head Start to policies mandating the dropout age, class size, and the length of the school day and school year to policies on the availability of affordable college education for all who wish to pursue higher education. Every educational policy and program proposal should be considered in light of its mental health impacts. Improving education for all will improve the physical health and mental health of current and future generations.

Key Points

- Better schooling leads to higher wages in better jobs and thus better living conditions, enhanced productivity and earnings, improved interpersonal relationships, better parenting, greater social connections, and improved quality of life. These positive factors lead to healthier food choices, better medical care, and improved health status. Better education is clearly linked to better mental health and a lower risk for behavioral disorders.

- The school is an environment in which youths learn social skills, values, the meaning of usefulness and work, self-regulation and control, frustration tolerance, and many other psychological and social skills, all of which support mental health.

- Achieving excellence in education requires a combination of many factors, including a safe and healthy school setting, caring and effective school administrators, good teachers with sufficient support systems and wages, and small class sizes.

- Preschool programs that institute the High/Scope Perry Preschool model have shown that high-quality early childhood education programs for young children living in poverty improve their intellectual and social development in childhood, as well as their school success, economic performance, and other social and health outcomes in adulthood. The home literacy environment also represents an arena for intervention during the preschool years.

- Decreasing students' dropout rates and encouraging high school graduation affect future educational and employment trajectories and are relevant to promoting both physical and mental health.

References

Adler NE, Rehkopf DH: U.S. disparities in health: descriptions, causes, and mechanisms. Annu Rev Public Health 29:235–252, 2008 18031225

Adler NE, Boyce T, Chesney MA, et al: Socioeconomic status and health. The challenge of the gradient. Am Psychol 49(1):15–24, 1994 8122813

Aikens NL, Barbarin O: Socioeconomic differences in reading trajectories: the contribution of family, neighborhood, and school contexts. J Educ Psychol 100:235–251, 2008

Betts JR, Tang YE: The Effect of Charter Schools on Student Achievement: A Meta-Analysis of the Literature. Bothell, University of Washington, 2011. Available at: http://files.eric.ed.gov/fulltext/ED526353.pdf. Accessed April 18, 2014.

Bifulco R, Ladd HF: The impacts of charter schools on student achievement: evidence from North Carolina. Education Finance and Policy 1:50–90, 2006

Case A, Lubotsky D, Paxson C: Economic status and health in childhood: the origins of the gradient. Am Econ Rev 92(5):1308–1334, 2002

Cohen AK, Syme SL: Education: a missed opportunity for public health intervention. Am J Public Health 103(6):997–1001, 2013 23597373

Cook JA, Solomon ML: The Community Scholar Program: an outcome study of supported education for students with severe mental illness. Psychosocial Rehabilitation Journal 17:83–97, 1993

Dohrenwend BS, Dohrenwend BP: Class and race as status-related sources of stress, in Social Stress. Edited by Levine S, Scotch NA. Chicago, IL, Aldine Transaction, 1973, pp 111–140

Economist Intelligence Unit: The Learning Curve. London, Pearson Education, 2014. Available at: http://thelearningcurve.pearson.com. Accessed April 18, 2014.

Frede EC: The role of program quality in producing early childhood program benefits. Future Child 5(3):115–132, 1995 8835517

Freudenberg N, Ruglis J: Reframing school dropout as a public health issue. Prev Chronic Dis 4(4):A107, 2007 17875251

Galea S, Tracy M, Hoggatt KJ, et al: Estimated deaths attributable to social factors in the United States. Am J Public Health 101(8):1456–1465, 2011 21680937

Gormley WT, Phillips D, Adelstein S, et al: Head Start's comparative advantage: myth or reality. Policy Stud J 38(3):397–418, 2010

Goosby BJ: Early life course pathways of adult depression and chronic pain. J Health Soc Behav 54(1):75–91, 2013 23426854

Hanushek EA, Peterson PE, Woessmann L: Achievement Growth: International and U.S. State Trends in Student Performance. Cambridge, MA, Harvard's Program on Education Policy and Governance & Education Next, 2012. Available at: http://www.hks.harvard.edu/pepg/PDF/Papers/PEPG12-03_CatchingUp.pdf. Accessed April 18, 2014.

Hoffman FL, Mastrianni X: The role of supported education in the inpatient treatment of young adults: a two-site comparison. Psychosocial Rehabilitation Journal 17:109–119, 1993

Hyun JK, Quinn BC, Madon T, et al: Graduate student mental health: needs assessment and utilization of counseling services. Journal of College Student Development 47:247–266, 2006

Kaneko Y, Motohashi Y: Male gender and low education with poor mental health literacy: a population-based study. J Epidemiol 17(4):114–119, 2007 17641446

Kitzrow MA: The mental health needs of today's college students: challenges and recommendations. NASPA Journal 41:167–181, 2003

Matthews KA, Gallo LC: Psychological perspectives on pathways linking socioeconomic status and physical health. Annu Rev Psychol 62:501–530, 2011 20636127

McEwen BS, Seeman T: Protective and damaging effects of mediators of stress. Elaborating and testing the concepts of allostasis and allostatic load. Ann N Y Acad Sci 896:30–47, 1999 10681886

Miron G, Nelson C: Student achievement in charter schools: what we know and why we know so little, in Taking Account of Charter Schools: What's Happened and What's Next? Edited by Bulkley KE, Wohlstetter P. New York, Teachers College Press, 2004, pp 161–175

Muennig P, Woolf SH: Health and economic benefits of reducing the number of students per classroom in US primary schools. Am J Public Health 97(11):2020–2027, 2007 17901430

Patel V: Mental health in low- and middle-income countries. Br Med Bull 81–82:81–96, 2007 17470476

Perkins SC, Finegood ED, Swain JE: Poverty and language development: roles of parenting and stress. Innov Clin Neurosci 10(4):10–19, 2013 23696954

Ruberman W, Weinblatt E, Goldberg JD, et al: Psychosocial influences on mortality after myocardial infarction. N Engl J Med 311(9):552–559, 1984 6749228

Sass TR: Charter schools and student achievement in Florida. Education Finance and Policy 1:91–122, 2006

Schulman K: Policy Report: Overlooked Benefits of Prekindergarten. New Brunswick, NJ, National Institute for Early Education Research, 2005. Available at: http://nieer.org/resources/policyreports/report6.pdf. Accessed April 14, 2014.

Schweinhart LJ, Montie J, Xiang Z, et al: The High/Scope Perry Preschool Study Through Age 40: Summary, Conclusions, and Frequently Asked Questions. Ypsilanti, MI, HighScope Educational Research Foundation, 2005, pp 194–215

Seeman TE, McEwen BS, Rowe JW, et al: Allostatic load as a marker of cumulative biological risk: MacArthur studies of successful aging. Proc Natl Acad Sci USA 98(8):4770–4775, 2001 11287659

Substance Abuse and Mental Health Services Administration: Supported Education Evidence-Based Practices (EBP) Kit. Rockville, MD, Substance Abuse and Mental Health Services Administration, 2012. Available at: http://store.samhsa.gov/product/Supported-Education-Evidence-Based-Practices-EBP-Kit/SMA11-4654CD-ROM. Accessed April 18, 2014.

Unger KV, Anthony WA, Sciarappa K, et al: A supported education program for young adults with long-term mental illness. Hosp Community Psychiatry 42(8):838–842, 1991 1894260

Williams LK, Andrianopoulos N, Cleland V, et al: Associations between education and personal income with body mass index among Australian women
   residing in disadvantaged neighborhoods. Am J Health Promot 28(1):59–65,
   2013 23458372
Zimmer R, Buddin R: Charter school performance in two large urban districts.
   J Urban Econ 60:307–326, 2006

5

Unemployment, Underemployment, and Job Insecurity

Brian S. McGregor, Ph.D.
Kisha B. Holden, Ph.D., M.S.C.R.

If a man doesn't have a job or an income, he has neither life nor liberty nor the possibility for the pursuit of happiness. He merely exists.

Martin Luther King Jr., 1929–1968

A fundamental human right inherent to individual responsibility and self-preservation is the ability to be self-sufficient and provide for one's basic needs. Unfortunately, many individuals and families in the United States struggle to attain this basic human right. This struggle is in part because of the complexities of unemployment, underemployment, job insecurity, and other deleterious sociocultural and environmental ills that damage many of our communities. The reality is quite disconcerting, particularly in a country that boasts an economy that leads the world in resources, perceived financial stability, and opportunities to achieve the American Dream.

The recent economic downturn and subsequent Great Recession in the United States led to double-digit unemployment rates, which had not been seen since the recession of the early 1980s. As a result, large numbers of individuals have been plagued by long-term unemployment, underemployment, and job insecurity. Specific groups are vulnerable to particularly high rates of unemployment compared with other population groups, especially individuals of black, Hispanic, American Indian, and Alaska Native race or ethnicity (Bureau of Labor Statistics 2014a).

Being gainfully employed—being able to fully support oneself and one's family—is an essential part of success in modern life. Unemployment and unstable or insecure employment are associated with poor physical and mental health outcomes across a variety of populations and conditions. In addition to having a job, a person's rank in his or her job is also relevant to physical and emotional health. The groundbreaking Whitehall study described the social gradient in health that exists among British civil servants on the basis of employment grade (Marmot et al. 1991). Thus, working not only to improve employment opportunities but also to enhance working conditions among the employed will improve the health of the nation. In considering the social determinants of mental health, we will consider the ways that unemployment, underemployment, and job insecurity contribute to poor mental health and increase risk for (and worsen the course of) mental illnesses.

Employment Insecurity: An Overview

Key Definitions: Unemployment, Underemployment, and Job Insecurity

According to the Bureau of Labor Statistics (2014b), unemployed individuals are defined as those persons who "do not have a job, have actively looked for work in the prior four weeks, and are currently available for work." Actively looking for work may consist of any of the following activities: contacting an employer directly or having a job interview; getting in touch with a public or private employment agency, friends, or relatives about getting a job; contacting a school or university employment center; sending out resumes or completing job applications; placing or answering job advertisements; checking union or professional registers; and engaging in some other means of active job search. The unemployment rate does not fully encompass all those without work—the Bureau of Labor Statistics also measures *discouraged workers*, who are unemployed and have not sought work in the past 4 weeks because they specifically believe that there are no jobs available for them. They also consider *marginally attached workers*, who also have not sought work for any other reason. These individuals are not directly included in the calculated unemployment rate (Bureau of Labor Statistics 2014b).

Underemployment is a measure of employment and labor utilization that represents how well the labor force is being utilized in terms of skills, experience, and availability to work. At the individual level, the underemployment classification includes workers who are highly skilled but work in low-paying jobs, workers who are highly skilled but work in low-skill jobs, and part-time workers who would prefer to be working full time but give economic reasons for part-time work (Bureau of Labor Statistics 2014b). Underemployment differs from unemployment in that the individual is working, although not at his or her full capabilities.

Job insecurity, at the individual level, refers to a state of uncertainty held by an individual who feels as if his or her job is in a constant state of jeopardy as a result of an unsteady economic or industrial climate. Within this classification, individuals are employed; however, they are unsure if their current employment status is safe or stable when regularly faced with mass layoffs and/or closings within their industry. Unlike unemployment or underemployment, job insecurity refers to an internal experience and leaves the individual without clear relief options and structural supports, which makes coping with this experience challenging (Burgard et al. 2009).

The labor force participation rate is another important measure pertaining to the U.S. workforce. The labor force is defined as the number of people in the United States who are working or are unemployed but available for work. The labor force participation rate refers to the percentage of working-age people (the civilian, noninstitutional population) who are either working or searching for work. When considered in conjunction with the unemployment rate, this rate is a key measure of the health of the labor market.

Prevalence of Unemployment and Underemployment in the United States

According to the U.S. Department of Labor, in March 2014, approximately 10.5 million Americans were unemployed, and the overall unemployment rate was 6.7%. However, the unemployment rate was significantly higher for blacks (12.1%) and Hispanics (8.1%) compared with non-Hispanic whites (5.9%) and Asians (5.4%), indicating ongoing employment inequalities for specific ethnic minority populations (Bureau of Labor Statistics 2014a). Because of demographic trends toward more retired and older adults, the recent economic recession, and a long-term decline of women in the workforce (after a rapid increase in the second half of the twentieth century), the labor force participation rate has been decreasing for many years and is currently 63.1%, which is considered low by historical standards (Bureau of Labor Statistics 2014a).

Unemployment, Underemployment, and Job Insecurity as Social Determinants of Health

Unemployment is clearly linked to poorer health. For example, research has identified relationships between unemployment and sleep disturbances, high serum cholesterol levels, and risk factors for cardiovascular disease among middle-aged men (Mattiasson et al. 1990). Such findings substantiate the long-standing observation of excessive mortality due to cardiovascular disease in countries with high rates of unemployment (Brenner 1987). Additional studies have uncovered associations between unemployment and elevated blood pressure and cholesterol (Weber and Lehnert 1997).

On the population level, plant closures and mass layoffs can lead to marked physical health impacts. A study of a community sample of high-unemployment census tracts in Michigan found higher self-reports of physical illness among the unemployed (Kessler et al. 1988). Furthermore, research suggests a cumulative effect of multiple job losses on risk for myocardial infarction (Dupre et al. 2012). As discussed by Gallo (2012), extensive research supports the many physical and mental health effects of unemployment (Table 5–1).

Clear associations between physical health and underemployment also exist. Individuals who are underemployed in terms of lower income have poorer functional physical health ratings, whereas those who are underemployed in terms of lower job status have poorer functional health and a greater prevalence of chronic diseases compared with appropriately employed individuals (Friedland and Price 2003).

Many studies have documented the adverse effects of job insecurity on health outcomes (McDonough 2000; Sverke et al. 2002). Perceived job insecurity is an important predictor of poorer self-rated health, with job-insecure workers more likely to report fair or poor self-rated health than secure workers (Burgard et al. 2009, 2012).

Unemployment, Underemployment, and Job Insecurity as Social Determinants of Mental Health

For decades, the fact that employment insecurity increases one's risk not only for physical health problems but also for behavioral disorders has been well documented, particularly in other industrialized countries (McKee-Ryan et al. 2005; Moynihan 2012; Paul and Moser 2006; Uutela

TABLE 5–1. Overall health status and number of physically and mentally unhealthy days in past 30 days among adults ages 18–64 years by employment status

Health status	Unemployed >1 year		Unemployed <1 year		Employed[a]	
	Percentage	95% CI	Percentage	95% CI	Percentage	95% CI
Overall health status						
Excellent or very good	39.7	38.1–41.4	49.2	47.7–51.2	52.7	62.2–63.1
Good	35.1	33.5–36.7	33.9	32.3–35.6	29.1	28.7–29.5
Fair or poor	25.2	23.8–26.7	16.6	15.4–18.0	8.2	8.0–8.5
Number of physically unhealthy days in past 30 days						
0	55.9	54.2–57.5	63.1	61.4–64.9	70.3	69.9–70.7
1–15	31.4	29.8–33.0	28.6	27.0–30.2	26.1	25.7–26.5
16–30	12.8	11.7–13.9	8.3	7.3–9.4	3.6	3.5–3.8
Number of mentally unhealthy days in past 30 days						
0	50.6	48.9–52.3	54.2	52.4–56.0	67.3	66.9–67.8
1–15	32.6	31.0–34.3	32.9	31.2–34.6	27.3	26.8–27.7
16–30	16.8	15.6–18.1	12.9	11.9–14.1	5.4	5.2–5.6

Note. 95% CI=95% confidence interval.
[a]Employed for wages or self-employed.
Source. Modified from Centers for Disease Control and Prevention 2013

2010). In fact, research that characterizes unemployment, underemployment, and job insecurity as social determinants of mental health may be more robust than the evidence for the impact of these factors on physical health. Furthermore, these employment-related variables have been linked to a wide variety of markers of poor mental health, including psychological distress, depression, anxiety, psychosomatic symptoms, poor self-esteem, and self-reported poor mental health (Paul and Moser 2009).

Impact of Unemployment on Mental Health

Several studies have examined the relationship between employment status and the occurrence of behavioral disorders. The most common conceptualizations apply stress and coping theory and treat unemployment as an undesirable life event that challenges an individual's adaptive capacity. This idea is based on the latent deprivation model, which hypothesizes that the cause of mental health problems among those who are unemployed is related to the lack of five latent functions of employment (time structure, social contact, collective purpose, status, and activity), each of which is associated with important psychological needs (Jahoda 1982). As expected, the financial strain resulting from income loss has been identified as one driver of adverse mental health outcomes related to unemployment (Kessler et al. 1988). Furthermore, loss of employment can lead to loss of employer-based health insurance benefits, which limits access and ability to afford care, especially for people with existing mental illnesses (Melfi et al. 1999).

In-depth study of four General Motors plant closures in the United States in 1987 yielded several analyses highlighting the deleterious mental health effects (including depression, anxiety, and somatization) in those communities, particularly among minority and less educated population groups (Broman et al. 1990, 1995; Hamilton et al. 1990, 1993). More recent studies have confirmed the association between employment status and mental health and substance use disorders. In an extensive meta-analysis, McKee-Ryan et al. (2005) found evidence for a causal relationship between unemployment and poor mental health. Specifically, cross-sectional studies found significant differences between employed and unemployed persons with regard to mental health, and longitudinal studies observed that job loss was associated with a statistically significant increase in distress symptoms (whereas finding a new job was associated with a statistically significant reduction in distress). However, Butterworth and colleagues (2012) found that the quality of the job was meaningful, in that individuals with the poorest-quality jobs had an equal number of or more mental health problems than unemployed individuals.

Studies have also found associations between unemployment and alcohol use disorders, although results are inconsistent (Catalano et al. 1993; Forcier 1988; Winton et al. 1986). Although some studies have noted a decrease in alcohol consumption among unemployed persons, which is often attributed to less income (Ettner 1997), others show an increase in alcohol use disorders associated with unemployment (Mulia et al. 2014). Yet another study found that the association varies significantly with duration of unemployment, with the recently unemployed drinking less than employed workers and the long-term unemployed drinking more (Khan et al. 2002). Additionally, there is ongoing debate about whether alcohol use disorders cause unemployment or whether unemployment leads to alcohol misuse (Dooley et al. 1992; Mullahy and Sindelar 1996), although both directions of causality are most likely at play.

Analyses have also focused on the existing high unemployment rates in the United States in specific population groups. Evaluation of various groups based on sex, age, race/ethnicity, and educational level consistently found an association between unemployment status and poor mental health across many diverse population groups (Mandal et al. 2011; Rosenthal et al. 2012). Collectively, these findings demonstrate that the negative impact of unemployment affects everyone but that special consideration should be given to the most vulnerable populations by tailoring appropriate interventions that address unemployment-related poor behavioral health outcomes among high-risk groups.

In analyzing the mental health consequences of unemployment, underemployment, and job insecurity, one must also consider the long-standing association between work status and suicide. In the United States, an increasing unemployment rate has been directly correlated with a rise in the overall suicide rate (Reeves et al. 2012). Similarly, studies have consistently demonstrated strong associations between suicide and unemployment in other countries (Blakely et al. 2003; Lewis and Sloggett 1998; Morrell et al. 1993). Causal pathways through which unemployment or job loss lead to increased suicide attempts are an area of recent interest. Classen and Dunn (2012) found that periods of unemployment longer than 5 weeks are positively associated with increased suicide risk for both men and women, especially between 15 and 26 weeks of unemployment. Additionally, they found an association between mass layoffs and increased suicide risk, potentially as a result of lack of future job prospects and loss of social networks (Classen and Dunn 2012).

Impact of Underemployment on Mental Health

Research describing the relationship between underemployment and mental health is limited because underemployment, or inadequate employment, has been studied less than unemployment (Dooley 2003). However, underemployment is directly associated with psychological distress and depression (Friedland and Price 2003; Herzog et al. 1991; Jones-Johnson and Johnson 1992).

Transitioning from adequate employment to underemployment can have mental health effects on individuals that are similar to those that result from becoming unemployed. As discussed in the section "Impact of Unemployment on Mental Health," the quality of employment is as important as whether or not an individual is employed. Underemployed individuals in poor-quality jobs may have rates of mental distress that are similar to or greater than those of unemployed people, perhaps because of the increased uncertainty that is often associated with underemployment. Individuals appear to have more difficulty coping with issues related to underemployment compared with unemployment, possibly because of job insecurity, low job satisfaction, and disrupted relationships with coworkers (Burgard et al. 2009; Dooley 2003).

Job Insecurity and Mental Health Outcomes

Job insecurity has far-reaching, complex consequences (Figure 5–1). A critical question is how macrolevel conditions, such as high or rising levels of unemployment, translate directly into individual-level, subjective feelings of insecurity.

Some studies find strong evidence to support an association between job insecurity and poor mental health (Cheng and Chan 2008; Larson et al. 1994; Sverke et al. 2002), whereas others note a moderate relationship between psychological distress and job insecurity (De Witte 1999; Silla et al. 2008) or report no association at all (Fox and Chancey 1998). Additional research is needed to clarify the relationship between job insecurity and poor mental health and mental illnesses.

Employment Insecurity in the Clinical Setting

Stress and coping theory suggests that addressing stressors (e.g., job loss, impoverished neighborhoods, and lack of educational opportunities) and identifying positive coping mechanisms (e.g., social support networks and engaging in healthy behaviors) may improve one's outlook and outcome concerning personal challenges (Krohne 2001). Thus, it is critical that mental health providers explore strategies for reducing stress

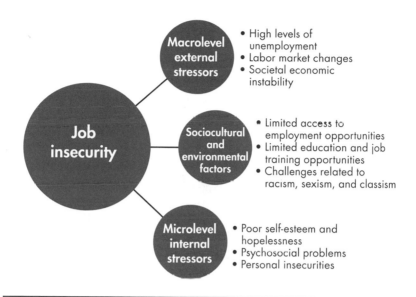

FIGURE 5–1.   Multilevel factors associated with job insecurity.

and improving positive coping among patients at risk for unemployment or underemployment. Once employment is secured, strategies must be in place to support individuals' maintenance of employment, achievement of goals, and coping with uncertainties inherent in the job market.

Case Example: The Hard Work of Managing a Serious Mental Illness and Unemployment

Marcus Stephenson is a 36-year-old black male who does not have a permanent address and lives with various family members and friends for brief periods of time. He was diagnosed with diabetes during childhood, and over the years he has had difficulty managing his illness because of repeated episodes of homelessness. Mr. Stephenson was in a convenience store when he became confused and agitated. He reported blurred vision and became combative with employees and customers in the store. Law enforcement was called, and when officers arrived, they noticed that he appeared malnourished and disheveled and that he was wearing a bracelet indicating that he has diabetes. They called an ambulance, and paramedics stabilized Mr. Stephenson and transported him to the local emergency department.

Staff at the emergency department stabilized Mr. Stephenson's symptoms associated with diabetes, but he remained agitated and combative. Dr. John Sullivan, the on-call psychiatrist, was asked to evaluate Mr. Stephenson. After a brief evaluation, Dr. Sullivan admitted Mr. Stephenson to the crisis stabilization unit. After administering psychotropic medications to help stabilize Mr. Stephenson's agitation and combativeness, Dr. Sullivan spoke with him. Still quite angry, Mr. Stephenson told Dr. Sullivan that he knows he was diagnosed with schizophrenia but refuses to take any medications because they make him feel "weird" and he cannot function as he wants to. Mr. Stephenson said he hears the medical staff laughing at him all the time and that they don't really want to help him.

The following day, the crisis stabilization treatment team meets with Mr. Stephenson. During their assessment, they gather information about his current living situation, relationships with family, the impact of diabetes on his life, and employment. They learn from Mr. Stephenson that he has tenuous relationships with his younger brother and older sister and has had very little contact with other relatives. He gets around on public transportation when he has the money. Mr. Stephenson tells the team that he enjoys writing and reciting poetry on occasion. His employment history includes working as a bartender in several restaurants but rarely ever full time or for longer than 1 year. When Dr. Sullivan mentions the idea of medications, Mr. Stephenson becomes angry again and insists that they tell him the "real reason" why they want him to take medications. However, during the treatment team meeting, Mr. Stephenson does agree to speak with Manny Ramos, a psychosocial rehabilitation specialist, later in the day.

When Mr. Ramos meets with Mr. Stephenson, he finds out that right after high school Mr. Stephenson attended community college for engineering studies and had been interested in becoming an air force pilot. Mr. Stephenson describes his skills in math, physics, and computer science as above average. However, he did not finish community college and has been on his own, largely unemployed, ever since. Mr. Stephenson was able to pay for most of his expenses by working part time as a bartender at various restaurants, lounges, and clubs whenever he was notified of jobs by a few bartender friends. These opportunities declined significantly in 2008 during the recession, but Mr. Stephenson tells Mr. Ramos that the reason was mostly because the owners and other bartenders at multiple businesses plotted against him because he was making too much money. Mr. Stephenson says that he does not want a formal job because he knows he will lose the Social Security Disability Insurance (SSDI) for which he was recently approved. However, Mr. Stephenson also indicates that he would like to be a waiter in a fine-dining restaurant, which would give him the opportunity to relate to his coworkers and put him in a setting where he can interact with strangers, something he had enjoyed as a bartender. When Mr. Ramos tries to explain that there is flexibility with SSDI that will allow him some employment opportunities, Mr. Stephenson interrupts him and tells Mr. Ramos that others have tried to get him to lose his SSDI and that he will not allow him to do that. Mr. Ramos sets another appointment to continue the consultation with Mr. Stephenson.

Mr. Stephenson presents several familiar challenges to Mr. Ramos and the other members of the treatment team. He clearly has employable skills and wants to work, but he presents with several barriers to obtaining and maintaining a job, perhaps the most prominent of which are his medical and psychiatric conditions. Currently, a job as a bartender is not one that he can rely on or consistently perform well given his mental health issues. Although Mr. Stephenson clearly values working as a bartender or waiter, it could affect his mental health in undesired ways, including having to work late-night shifts. The health care system has many challenges in working with Mr. Stephenson to manage both his health and employment challenges.

Assessing Employment Insecurity and Related Risk Factors in the Clinical Setting

The potential emotional, psychosocial, cognitive, and material benefits to patients when their clinicians support employment goals are significant, and this support should be a routine part of clinical practice. Mental health professionals can engage patients in discussions about employment-related issues, including unemployment and related distress, underemployment, poor motivation to work, and job insecurity. In addition, clinicians can assess the impact of unemployment on partner intimacy, friendships, and social status. Patients may not immediately recognize the significance of employment status on their identity, self-esteem, relationships, and community participation. Cultural competence is also a necessary skill for providers because an individual's membership within subgroups (including those pertaining to race/ethnicity, sexual orientation, and immigration, to name a few) may also have an impact on their experience of job loss and related distress. Exploring a patient's work history and alternative employable skills may be an important pathway to reduced psychological distress and clarity around future employment goals.

Understanding the multiple impacts that job insecurity, underemployment, and unemployment have on the individual may lead to changes in therapeutic goals. Exploring these topics with patients can be an important aspect of planning treatment goals. Patients may decide to become entrepreneurs, to make child rearing their priority, to pursue educational goals, or to switch their careers. This process can vary on the basis of how long the individual is out of work, other sources of distress, and financial stability during the period of unemployment.

How Clinicians Can Address Unemployment and Underemployment in the Clinical Setting

An increased understanding of unemployment as a social determinant of mental health should lead to greater focus on issues such as unemployment and underemployment during clinicians' encounters with patients. Mental health professionals can assist patients in developing realistic and achievable work-related goals and monitoring progress toward goal attainment. They can become familiar with services and resources pertaining to work readiness, psychosocial rehabilitation, vocational rehabilitation, job skills programs, and supported employment programs. Clinicians can support their clients' sense of self-efficacy and motivation toward achieving short- and long-term employment goals that will potentially bring tangible benefits, including increased job security and financial stability.

Although psychiatric institutions may have been the birthplace of vocational rehabilitation services, such services have increasingly come to be located in community settings where specialists provide a range of occupational and work therapies to mental health consumers seeking employment (Rössler 2006; Wanberg 2012). Several approaches are used to assist individuals with preparing for work, including strategies that focus on providing unemployed individuals with knowledge and skills for work.

One evidence-based practice is supported employment, which gives mental health consumers opportunities in competitive employment and provides them with the support needed to perform well in the job (Drake et al. 2012). The Dartmouth Individual Placement and Support (IPS) Supported Employment Center has been at the forefront of improving employment for people with serious mental illnesses using this model. As shown in Figure 5–2, IPS supported employment has proven to be cost-effective and has improved mental health and well-being over time (Bond et al. 2012).

Policy Approaches to Unemployment, Underemployment, and Job Insecurity as Social Determinants of Mental Health

State Programs Affecting Unemployment and Underemployment

Each state has policy initiatives to address unemployment among its residents. The approaches that each state undertakes are, in part, a reflection of the challenges each faces and the political will within the pop-

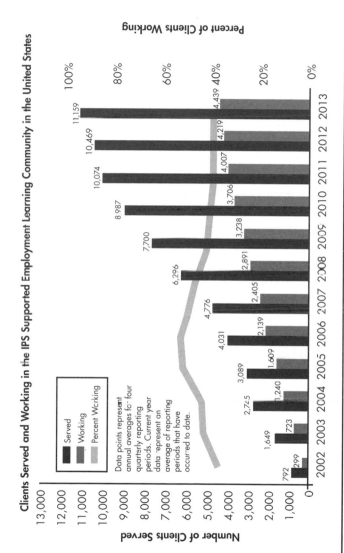

FIGURE 5–2. Impact of the Dartmouth Individual Placement and Support (IPS) supported employment program.

Source. Modified from Bob Drake, PowerPoint presentation, Dartmouth Psychiatric Research Center, Lebanon, NH. Available at http://sites.dartmouth.edu/IPS/j-j-dartmouth-community-mental-health-program. Accessed December 1, 2013.

ulace to take on issues related to employment. The seasonally adjusted February 2014 unemployment rates among the states ranged from a low of 2.6% in North Dakota to a high of 9.0% in Rhode Island (Bureau of Labor Statistics 2014c). Thus, there is great variation among states in both the severity of the issues associated with unemployment and solutions to address these issues.

Some states have developed policy and programmatic strategies that reflect an understanding and awareness of the relationship between mental health and employment insecurity. For example, researchers at the Michigan Prevention Research Center designed and evaluated the Job Opportunities and Basic Skills Training (JOBS) program to assist unemployed workers with becoming reemployed and to effectively cope with the emotional and psychosocial stressors associated with unemployment and job searching. Individuals, particularly women and those with less education, who participated in the JOBS program had lower levels of depression and obtained higher-paying jobs (Price et al. 1992; Vinokur et al. 1991). This program demonstrates the benefits of not only strengthening the employability of individuals but also using resources to assist individuals in coping with unemployment. The JOBS program has been successfully implemented in other states, including Maryland and California.

Unemployment insurance benefits provide a percentage of previous pay to newly unemployed workers, delivering temporary financial assistance while recipients look for work. Unemployment insurance is a joint federal-state program, with a high degree of flexibility given to states to administer the program. Unemployment compensation benefits often help to partly alleviate the stress and uncertainty associated with unemployment and may also buffer against some of the anxiety associated with job insecurity. The benefits of unemployment insurance are the subject of ongoing debate, but evidence exists to support lower rates of depression among unemployed individuals receiving unemployment compensation compared with unemployed individuals who do not receive benefits (Rodriguez et al. 1997). Similar findings have been observed in analyses among countries, with those with generous unemployment benefits having fewer negative mental health effects associated with unemployment than countries with weaker benefits (Paul and Moser 2009).

Federal Policy and Programs Affecting Unemployment and Underemployment

Specific policies and laws set forth by the federal government have attempted to address the negative effects of unemployment. The Personal Responsibility and Work Opportunity Reconciliation Act of 1996, which established Temporary Assistance for Needy Families (TANF), had important implications for unemployed and poor individuals because it included a workforce development component as a necessary condition to receive welfare benefits. Welfare recipients are at higher risk for mental health problems (Danziger et al. 2000); however, a causal relationship between employment and mental health is not well established. Nevertheless, it is important to consider employment barriers associated with mental illnesses and to improve access to treatment for those individuals receiving welfare benefits.

The Fair Labor Standards Act (FLSA) and the Family and Medical Leave Act (FMLA) aim to set fair workplace environments and wage standards and protect workers to ensure employment stability. Debate over the importance of paying people a "living wage" could lead to an increase in the minimum wage, which is set by the FLSA. Job and skills training programs also exist to increase the number of skilled workers in the United States, which could give people the opportunity to seek higher-wage, higher-quality jobs. The Organisation for Economic Co-operation and Development (2012) promotes skills development through policy interventions as an effective methodology to decrease unemployment.

Both men and women with criminal records have a high level of unemployment and underemployment. Given the "criminalization" of mental illnesses, it is important to consider opportunities for rehabilitation and employment among individuals recently released from jails and prisons. The Legal Action Center (2004) has developed a report on state legal barriers faced by people with criminal records, including employment barriers. The Legal Action Center found multiple employment barriers in many states, including laws that permit employers and licensing agencies to consider arrests that never led to convictions in employment decisions, as well as laws that permit employers to deny jobs to or fire anyone with a criminal record without consideration of individual history or circumstance. "Ban the Box" campaigns advocate for removing the question on job applications that asks if the applicant has ever been convicted of a felony. National interest in reducing criminal justice recidivism is increasing, and employment and housing are at the forefront of this discussion.

If the health care system in this country is expected to place greater emphasis on prevention, health promotion, and wellness, increased focus on two main areas is warranted. First, more rigorous investigations are needed to find strategies to assist individuals coping with job loss, unwanted delays in obtaining employment, unsatisfactory underemployment, and other undesired outcomes. Additionally, mental health professionals need to implement evidence-based interventions to help patients and their families navigate the employment-seeking landscape, such as supported employment.

Policy strategies to improve employment security for individuals diagnosed with a mental illness may be explored and developed within the context of public-sector insurance. In many states, Medicaid covers supported employment, which has a strong evidence base for improving employment among individuals with mental illnesses, particularly the IPS model. Greater advocacy is needed to encourage awareness and increase implementation of these services.

Promoting Healthful and Productive Employment: A Role for Everyone

Unemployment, underemployment, and job insecurity exact a significant economic, physical, and emotional toll on individuals, families, and communities. Gainful employment not only conveys financial resources for the individual with the job but also provides a sense of pride, belonging, and social support, which are crucial to an individual's well-being. The tangible and intangible benefits of fulfilling work are especially important to individuals diagnosed with mental illnesses who are pursuing recovery.

The literature on the impact of employment insecurity on mental health is unequivocal. However, action to support programs and policies that help address the negative impacts of unemployment, underemployment, and job insecurity lags behind the data. Behavioral health professionals have a responsibility to advocate for policies that improve and support suitable, stable employment for individual patients as well as the general population. A diverse group of stakeholders, including legislators, mental health professionals, governmental agencies, health care advocates, and others, must form cross-sector collaborations to enhance opportunities for fulfilling, meaningful work to improve the well-being of all Americans.

Key Points

- Extensive evidence supports the link between unemployment, underemployment, and job insecurity and poor mental health outcomes, including depressive disorders, anxiety disorders, alcohol use disorders, and suicide.

- Employment security and mental health and well-being have a bidirectional relationship, such that employment security promotes good mental health and individuals with good mental health are better able to seek, obtain, and maintain gainful employment.

- Subgroups including young workers, blacks, Hispanics, and immigrants have higher levels of unemployment and underemployment than other population groups.

- Although practice and policy strategies that strengthen employment and mental health outcomes exist, poor outcomes remain. Replication of studies and broader dissemination of high-fidelity, evidence-based programs are necessary to reduce psychological distress resulting from unemployment and underemployment and to increase employment security.

- Mental health providers have a responsibility to engage patients in a discussion about employment-related issues, including unemployment and related distress, underemployment, motivation to work, and job insecurity. They can also advocate for policies and programs that support employment opportunities and employment insurance benefits.

References

Blakely TA, Collings SCD, Atkinson J: Unemployment and suicide. Evidence for a causal association? J Epidemiol Community Health 57(8):594–600, 2003 12883065

Bond GR, Drake RE, Campbell K: The effectiveness of the individual placement and support model of supported employment for young adults: results from four randomized controlled trials. Paper presented at the International Early Psychosis Association, San Francisco, CA, 2012

Brenner MH: Economic change, alcohol consumption and heart disease mortality in nine industrialized countries. Soc Sci Med 25(2):119–132, 1987 3660003

Broman CL, Hamilton VL, Hoffman WS: Unemployment and its effects on families: evidence from a plant closing study. Am J Community Psychol 18(5):643–659, 1990

Broman CL, Hamilton VL, Hoffman WS, et al: Race, gender, and the response to stress: autoworkers' vulnerability to long-term unemployment. Am J Community Psychol 23(6):813–842, 1995 8638552

Bureau of Labor Statistics: Employment Situation Summary. Washington, DC, Bureau of Labor Statistics, 2014a. Available at: http://www.bls.gov/news.release/empsit.nr0.htm. Accessed April 13, 2014.

Bureau of Labor Statistics: Labor Force Characteristics from the Current Population Survey, Washington, DC, Bureau of Labor Statistics, 2014b. Available at: http://www.bls.gov/cps/lfcharacteristics.htm. Accessed April 14, 2014.

Bureau of Labor Statistics: Unemployment Rates for States. Washington, DC, Bureau of Labor Statistics, 2014c Available at: www.bls.gov/web/laus/laumstrk.htm. Accessed April 13, 2014.

Burgard SA, Brand JE, House JS: Perceived job insecurity and worker health in the United States. Soc Sci Med 69(5):777–785, 2009 19596166

Burgard SA, Kalousova L, Seefeldt KS: Perceived job insecurity and health: the Michigan Recession and Recovery Study. J Occup Environ Med 54(9):1101–1106, 2012 22929796

Butterworth P, Leach LS, Pirkis J, et al: Poor mental health influences risk and duration of unemployment: a prospective study. Soc Psychiatry Psychiatr Epidemiol 47(6):1013–1021, 2012 21681454

Catalano R, Dooley D, Wilson G, Hough R: Job loss and alcohol abuse: a test using data from the Epidemiologic Catchment Area project. J Health Soc Behav 34(3):215–225, 1993 7989666

Centers for Disease Control and Prevention: CDC health disparities and inequalities report, United States, 2013. MMWR 62(3)(suppl):1–187, 2013

Cheng GH-L, Chan DK-S: Who suffers more from job insecurity? A meta-analytic review. Appl Psychol 57(2):272–303, 2008

Classen TJ, Dunn RA: The effect of job loss and unemployment duration on suicide risk in the United States: a new look using mass-layoffs and unemployment duration. Health Econ 21(3):338–350, 2012 21322087

Danziger SK, Kalil A, Anderson NJ: Human capital, health and mental health of welfare recipients: co-occurrence and correlates. J Soc Issues 56(4):635–654, 2000

De Witte H: Job insecurity and psychological well-being: review of the literature and exploration of some unresolved issues. European Journal of Work and Organizational Psychology 8(2):155–177, 1999

Dooley D: Unemployment, underemployment, and mental health: conceptualizing employment status as a continuum. Am J Community Psychol 32(1–2):9–20, 2003 14570431

Dooley D, Catalano R, Hough R: Unemployment and alcohol disorder in 1910 and 1990: drift versus social causation. J Occup Organ Psychol 65(4):277–290, 1992

Drake RE, Bond GR, Becker DR: Individual Placement and Support: An Evidence-Based Approach to Supported Employment, 1st Edition. New York, Oxford University Press, 2012

Dupre ME, George LK, Liu G, et al: The cumulative effect of unemployment on risks for acute myocardial infarction. Arch Intern Med 172(22):1731–1737, 2012 23401888

Ettner SL: Measuring the human cost of a weak economy: does unemployment lead to alcohol abuse? Soc Sci Med 44(2):251–260, 1997 9015877

Forcier MW: Unemployment and alcohol abuse: a review. J Occup Med 30(3):246–251, 1988 3283302

Fox GL, Chancey D: Sources of economic distress: individual and family outcomes. J Fam Issues 19(6):725–749, 1998

Friedland DS, Price RH: Underemployment: consequences for the health and well-being of workers. Am J Community Psychol 32(1–2):33–45, 2003 14570433

Gallo WT: Evolution of research on the effect of unemployment on acute myocardial infarction risk. Arch Intern Med 172(22):1737–1738, 2012 23165943

Hamilton VL, Broman CL, Hoffman WS, et al: Hard times and vulnerable people: initial effects of plant closing on autoworkers' mental health. J Health Soc Behav 31(2):123–140, 1990 2102492

Hamilton VL, Hoffman WS, Broman CL, et al: Unemployment, distress, and coping: a panel study of autoworkers. J Pers Soc Psychol 65(2):234–247, 1993 8366419

Herzog AR, House JS, Morgan JN: Relation of work and retirement to health and well-being in older age. Psychol Aging 6(2):202–211, 1991 1863389

Jahoda M: Employment and Unemployment, 1st Edition. New York, Cambridge University Press, 1982

Jones-Johnson G, Johnson WR: Subjective underemployment and psychosocial stress: the role of perceived social and supervisor support. J Soc Psychol 132(1):11–21, 1992 1507871

Kessler RC, Turner JB, House JS: Effects of unemployment on health in a community survey: main, modifying, and mediating effects. J Soc Issues 44(4):69–85, 1988

Khan S, Murray RP, Barnes GE: A structural equation model of the effect of poverty and unemployment on alcohol abuse. Addict Behav 27(3):405–423, 2002 12118628

Krohne HW: Stress and coping theories. The International Encyclopedia of the Social and Behavioral Sciences 22:15163–15170, 2001

Larson JH, Wilson SM, Beley R: Impact of job insecurity on marital and family relationships. Fam Relat 43:138–143, 1994

Legal Action Center: After Prison: Roadblocks to Reentry: A Report on State Legal Barriers Facing People With Criminal Records. Washington, DC, 2004. Available at http://www.lac.org/roadblocks-to-reentry. Accessed February 14, 2014.

Lewis G, Sloggett A: Suicide, deprivation, and unemployment: record linkage study. BMJ 317(7168):1283–1286, 1998 9804714

Mandal B, Ayyagari P, Gallo WT: Job loss and depression: the role of subjective expectations. Soc Sci Med 72(4):576–583, 2011 21183267

Marmot MG, Smith GD, Stansfeld S, et al: Health inequalities among British civil servants: the Whitehall II study. Lancet 337(8754):1387–1393, 1991 1674771

Mattiasson I, Lindgärde F, Nilsson JA, et al: Threat of unemployment and cardiovascular risk factors: longitudinal study of quality of sleep and serum cholesterol concentrations in men threatened with redundancy. BMJ 301(6750):461–466, 1990 2207398

McDonough P: Job insecurity and health. Int J Health Serv 30(3):453–476, 2000 11109176

McKee-Ryan F, Song Z, Wanberg CR, et al: Psychological and physical well-being during unemployment: a meta-analytic study. J Appl Psychol 90(1):53–76, 2005 15641890

Melfi CA, Croghan TW, Hanna MP: Access to treatment for depression in a Medicaid population. J Health Care Poor Underserved 10(2):201–215, 1999 10224826

Morrell S, Taylor R, Quine S, et al: Suicide and unemployment in Australia 1907–1990. Soc Sci Med 36(6):749–756, 1993 8480219

Moynihan R: Job insecurity contributes to poor health. BMJ 345:e5183, 2012 22859778

Mulia N, Zemore SE, Murphy R, et al: Economic loss and alcohol consumption and problems during the 2008 to 2009 U.S. recession. Alcohol Clin Exp Res 38(4):1026–1034, 2014

Mullahy J, Sindelar J: Employment, unemployment, and problem drinking. J Health Econ 15(4):409–434, 1996 10164037

Organisation for Economic Co-operation and Development: Better Skills, Better Jobs, Better Lives: A Strategic Approach to Skills Policies. Paris, OECD Publishing, 2012. Available at http://dx.doi.org/10.1787/9789264177338-en. Accessed November 26, 2013.

Paul KI, Moser K: Incongruence as an explanation for the negative mental health effects of unemployment: meta-analytic evidence. J Occup Organ Psychol 79(4):595–621, 2006

Paul KI, Moser K: Unemployment impairs mental health: meta-analyses. J Vocat Behav 74(3):264–282, 2009

Price RH, Van Ryn M, Vinokur AD: Impact of a preventive job search intervention on the likelihood of depression among the unemployed. J Health Soc Behav 33(2):158–167, 1992 1619263

Reeves A, Stuckler D, McKee M, et al: Increase in state suicide rates in the USA during economic recession. Lancet 380(9856):1813–1814, 2012 23141814

Rodriguez E, Lasch K, Mead JP: The potential role of unemployment benefits in shaping the mental health impact of unemployment. Int J Health Serv 27(4):601–623, 1997 9399109

Rosenthal L, Carroll-Scott A, Earnshaw VA, et al: The importance of full-time work for urban adults' mental and physical health. Soc Sci Med 75(9):1692–1696, 2012 22858166

Rössler W: Psychiatric rehabilitation today: an overview. World Psychiatry 5(3):151–157, 2006 17139342

Silla I, Cuyper N, Gracia FJ, et al: Job insecurity and well-being: moderation by employability. J Happiness Stud 10(6):739–751, 2008

Sverke M, Hellgren J, Näswall K: No security: a meta-analysis and review of job insecurity and its consequences. J Occup Health Psychol 7(3):242–264, 2002 12148956

Uutela A: Economic crisis and mental health. Curr Opin Psychiatry 23(2):127–130, 2010 20087188

Vinokur AD, van Ryn M, Gramlich EM, Price RH: Long-term follow-up and benefit-cost analysis of the Jobs Program: a preventive intervention for the unemployed. J Appl Psychol 76(2):213–219, 1991 1905293

Wanberg CR: The individual experience of unemployment. Annu Rev Psychol 63:369–396, 2012 21721936

Weber A, Lehnert G: Unemployment and cardiovascular diseases: a causal relationship? Int Arch Occup Environ Health 70(3):153–160, 1997 9298397

Winton M, Heather N, Robertson I: Effects of unemployment on drinking behavior: a review of the relevant evidence. Int J Addict 21(12):1261–1283, 1986 3542847

6

Economic Inequality, Poverty, and Neighborhood Deprivation

Marc W. Manseau, M.D., M.P.H.

*What a devil art thou, Poverty! How many de-
sires—how many aspirations after goodness and
truth—how many noble thoughts, loving wishes
toward our fellows, beautiful imaginings thou hast
crushed under thy heel, without remorse or
pause!*

Walt Whitman, 1819–1892

The World Health Organization defines health as "a state of complete physical, mental and social well-being and not merely the absence of disease or infirmity" (World Health Organization 1948, p. 100). Because people must be able to participate in the economy of their community and society in order to obtain life- and health-sustaining goods and services (e.g., food, health care, education), having the income necessary to do so is vital to health. Furthermore, from Émile Durkheim to Amartya Sen, sociologists, philosophers, and economists have long recognized that economic deprivation is about much more than low income and limited purchasing power (Durkheim 1897/1951; Sen 1999). Rather, poverty can be thought of as social exclusion and deficits of opportunity in life. In order

The author thanks Kim Hopper, Ph.D., from the Nathan Kline Institute, Orangeburg, New York, for his helpful and thought-provoking edits, suggestions, and comments.

to create a sense of value and possibility in life, achieve a measure of productivity and meaning, and access social status and connectedness, individuals and communities must be fully integrated into a society's system of work, exchange, and worth. Therefore, economic factors are vital in accessing the material and social means necessary for physical and mental well-being. These economic factors make economic inequality an important driver of health inequality and economic deprivation a powerful social determinant of poor physical and mental health outcomes.

This chapter explores the economic factors of income inequality, individual and household poverty, and neighborhood deprivation as social determinants of mental health. After a discussion of important definitions, recent trends in the United States, and conceptual issues, we review the epidemiological research linking economic factors and mental health outcomes. Finally, the discussion turns to both clinical and policy approaches to breaking the links between economic social determinants and poor mental health. Some researchers have aptly criticized the field of social epidemiology as overly empirical and lacking a sound theoretical and contextual basis (Frohlich et al. 2001). Although we concede that such arguments have some validity, an in-depth historical and theoretical discussion of the political economy of health and disease is beyond the scope of this chapter, which mainly reviews the most relevant and current empirical literature on the role of economic inequality, poverty, and neighborhood deprivation in shaping poor mental health outcomes.

Poverty and Inequality: An Overview

Defining Inequality, Poverty, and Neighborhood Deprivation

Although economic inequality can be defined in multiple ways, social epidemiologists have focused largely on income inequality, which is most commonly measured using the Gini coefficient (GC), named after its developer, Corrado Gini. The GC uses a Lorenz curve (a graphical representation of wealth distribution) to calculate the extent to which the distribution of income in a population deviates from perfect equality. More concretely, it has often been interpreted as the proportion of total income in a population or geographic area that would have to be transferred to achieve complete equality. Using differences in taxable income between households, the GC has a theoretical range between 0 and 1. An international study conducted by the Organisation for Economic Co-operation and Development in the late 2000s that ranked

34 countries from most to least equal found that the United States was ranked thirty-first, with a GC of 0.38. This ranking is in contrast to those of the Scandinavian and Nordic nations, which were the most equal with GCs around 0.25 (Organisation for Economic Co-operation and Development 2012). Although income inequality is a key metric in health research, it is important to note that it fails to capture broader inequality in total goods and services consumed or in accumulated wealth.

Poverty can also be measured in various ways, including but not limited to income-based measures of absolute poverty or deprivation, relative poverty, and wealth deficits. One's income relative to the federal poverty level (FPL) is the most common metric in the United States, notwithstanding the facts that it ignores important aspects of relative poverty, such as local cost of living and economic inequality, and that it does not take into account the receipt of government services and spending on public insurance programs. The 2014 FPL for a family of four is $23,850, with *near poor* being defined as between 100% and 200% of the FPL (U.S. Department of Health and Human Services 2014).

For a host of complex and interrelated historical, political, and economic reasons, over the past six decades, poverty has become increasingly and disproportionately concentrated in poor, largely urban neighborhoods inhabited by racial/ethnic minority populations. A growing body of literature has focused on the myriad physical and mental health effects of geographically concentrated poverty. Measurement of neighborhood deprivation is, perhaps not surprisingly, a thorny matter, with conceptual problems ranging from what level of analysis to use (e.g., zip codes vs. census tracts vs. census blocks) to how to measure poverty or deprivation (Krieger et al. 2002). However, a common and straightforward measure is the *extreme poverty neighborhood*, defined as an area or neighborhood where more than 40% of households are living below the FPL (U.S. Department of Health and Human Services 2014). Less geographically concentrated poverty in rural and remote areas has received relatively little attention in the epidemiological literature, possibly because a smaller proportion of the total U.S. population lives outside of metropolitan areas. In many ways, one might assume that the problems associated with rural poverty would be the same as those associated with poverty in general. However, rural/remote poverty comes with a host of unique and important difficulties that may contribute to poorer mental health, such as social isolation, trends in substance abuse, limited infrastructure, and decreased access to employment opportunities and health care (Simmons et al. 2008; Smokowski et al. 2013).

Trends in Inequality and Poverty in the United States

Economic inequality and poverty have been growing in the United States since the 1970s. An increasing share of income and, to an even greater extent, wealth in the United States has gone to the top of the income distribution; for most of the population, earnings after health care costs are taken into account have barely kept pace with inflation (Piketty and Saez 2003). For instance, between 1979 and 2005, the top 1% of earners in the United States had an income growth of over 150%, whereas the bottom 40% of earners saw their incomes remain largely stagnant (Gould 2013). A recent report by the U.S. Census Bureau showed that these concerning trends have only accelerated since 2007 with the Great Recession and anemic recovery (DeNavas-Walt et al. 2013). The report revealed that between 2007 and 2012, real household median income declined 8%, whereas earnings for the wealthy increased, showing that the economic "recovery" existed only for top earners. As a result, in 2012, the highest-earning quintile of the U.S. population accumulated 51% of the total income, with 22% of total income going to the top 5% of earners, whereas the lowest-earning quintile of the population obtained only 3% of total income. With respect to such statistics, it is important to note that examining income in isolation does not adequately consider wealth, which is distributed even more unequally in the United States.

The U.S. Census Bureau report also addressed trends in poverty, revealing that 15% of Americans (46.5 million people) were living in poverty by the end of 2012, which is 2.5% higher than the poverty rate in 2007 and represents the highest prevalence of poverty since the Great Depression. Even more disturbing, the number and proportion of children living in poverty have been steadily increasing, leading to a "juvenilization" of poverty in the United States. In 2012, approximately 22% of children in the United States, or 16.1 million children, were living below the FPL, and almost 40% of children were either poor or near-poor (DeNavas-Walt et al. 2013). As discussed in the section "Inequality, Poverty, and Neighborhood Deprivation as Social Determinants of Mental Health," poverty in childhood is particularly toxic to mental health, making this trend especially alarming from a public health perspective.

Conceptual Issues Related to Inequality, Poverty, and Neighborhood Deprivation

Because understanding the relationships between broad economic phenomena operating at the societal level and individual mental health outcomes is a complex endeavor, it is important to explore some key conceptual issues before more closely examining findings from the literature. This discussion will serve to organize the exploration of the empirical research base and will guide thinking about opportunities for intervention.

First, it is important to draw a distinction between *social causation* and *social selection*. Social causation implies that factors such as inequality and poverty cause poor mental health outcomes, whereas social selection means that people with poor mental health or mental illnesses are more likely to become poor or move to poor neighborhoods. A hierarchy of evidence for proving causation is generally believed to exist. Ecological studies are considered to provide the weakest evidence for causation because of the *ecological fallacy*, which suggests that group-level findings cannot necessarily be applied to individual group members. Cross-sectional observational studies are also very limited in terms of assessing causation. Retrospective and especially prospective longitudinal studies can better establish temporality, which is necessary for causality. Randomized experiments are the strongest in terms of determining causation, but given inherent difficulties with randomizing complex social phenomena, natural experiments or quasi-experimental studies often represent the highest-quality study design that social epidemiologists can rely on. There are, however, caveats to this hierarchy. For instance, ecological studies may be best for studying truly area-level effects; richer data can often be obtained in cross-sectional studies; and it is difficult, unethical, or impossible to experimentally manipulate the social determinants of health.

Second, it is important to understand that economic factors operate simultaneously on multiple levels to influence mental health outcomes. Figure 6–1 depicts these levels and provides examples of important variables representing each level. The social determinants themselves are produced largely at the societal level. For instance, income inequality is caused by a combination of historical factors, macroeconomic trends, and policy decisions, such as fiscal and tax policy, as well as other forms of public resource management. Trends in inequality then drive the amount of deprivation in a society as well as demographic and geographic patterns of poverty. Once formed at the societal level, the economic social determinants operate within populations to produce risk, protective, and resilience factors for mental health outcomes in communities, neighborhoods, families, and individuals. Researchers using observational study designs are able to apply various statistical techniques, such as multilevel analysis, to account for the interplay between these levels, which allows simultaneous examination of individual- and group-level variables (Diez-Roux 2000). However, regardless of the statistical technique applied, the study design considerations remain paramount in establishing causality.

Finally, in order to identify opportunities for and appropriately target interventions toward the relationships between economic factors and mental health, it is important to understand mediating and moderating variables. A mediating variable *explains* the relationship between two other variables, such that including the mediator in an analysis reduces the observed relationship between the two associated variables. An example is the relationship between economic inequality and health observed across countries, which is mediated, or partially explained, by differences in societal-level social capital (Wilkinson 1992). A moderating variable, on the other hand, *changes* the relationship between two variables, such that the observed relationship between the two associated variables is different in magnitude or direction at different values of the moderator. An example is the relationship between poverty and child mental health, which is moderated by the age at which poverty begins, with poverty at an earlier age being more deleterious (McLoyd 1998).

Inequality, Poverty, and Neighborhood Deprivation as Social Determinants of Health

The literature on the relationships between economic factors and various physical health outcomes is vast and nuanced and has a storied and fascinating history going back decades; indeed, such work established the field of social epidemiology in the United States (Syme 2005). A comprehensive review, or even a well-informed discussion, of this body of work is well beyond the scope of this chapter. However, it is important to note that income inequality, individual poverty and socioeconomic status, and area-level poverty have all been associated variously and robustly with numerous physical health outcomes, including but not limited to adult mortality (Kondo et al. 2009) and life expectancy (Wilkinson 1992), infant mortality and other birth outcomes (Metcalfe et al. 2011), cardiovascular disease (Clark et al. 2009), and self-reported physical well-being (Kondo et al. 2009). These associations have been shown to be largely independent, replicable, and present at multiple levels of analysis using sophisticated statistical techniques, such as multilevel analysis and meta-analysis. The literature on economic factors as social determinants of physical health therefore provides a strong basis from which to explore the relationships between economic factors and mental health.

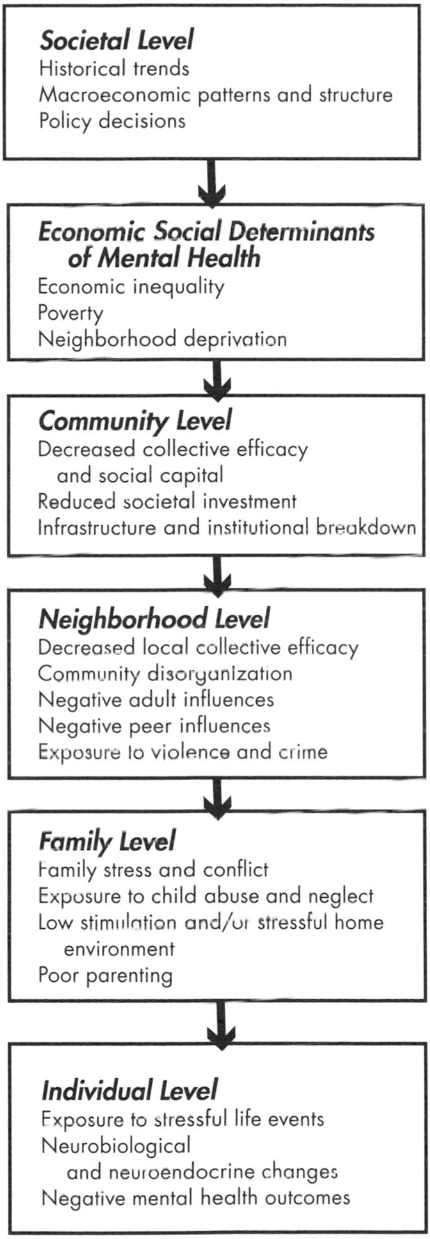

Societal Level
Historical trends
Macroeconomic patterns and structure
Policy decisions

**Economic Social Determinants
of Mental Health**
Economic inequality
Poverty
Neighborhood deprivation

Community Level
Decreased collective efficacy
    and social capital
Reduced societal investment
Infrastructure and institutional breakdown

Neighborhood Level
Decreased local collective efficacy
Community disorganization
Negative adult influences
Negative peer influences
Exposure to violence and crime

Family Level
Family stress and conflict
Exposure to child abuse and neglect
Low stimulation and/or stressful home
    environment
Poor parenting

Individual Level
Exposure to stressful life events
Neurobiological
    and neuroendocrine changes
Negative mental health outcomes

FIGURE 6–1.   Multiple levels of economic social determinants of mental health.

Inequality, Poverty, and Neighborhood Deprivation as Social Determinants of Mental Health

Figure 6–2 depicts variables mediating the effects of economic social determinants of mental health, and Figure 6–3 lists moderating variables. The relationships between area-level income inequality and mental health outcomes have been examined in observational studies both internationally and in the United States. At both county (Muramatsu 2003) and state (Messias et al. 2011; Pabayo et al. 2014) levels, income inequality has been independently associated with adult depression rates in the United States. Area-level income inequality has also been independently associated with adult outcomes ranging from self-reported poor mental health at the county level in a national sample (Zimmerman and Bell 2006) to drug overdose deaths in New York City (Nandi et al. 2006) to the incidence of schizophrenia in London, United Kingdom (Boydell et al. 2004). In an international study of 23 high-income countries (not including the United States), income inequality was robustly associated with an index of child well-being that included mental health problems, juvenile homicides, and poor childhood educational outcomes (Pickett and Wilkinson 2007). Various mediators of these relationships have been postulated, and some have been studied. These mediators include collective efficacy or social capital, most commonly defined as the degree of social cohesion and connectedness in a community (Sampson et al. 1997); investments in institutions, public services, and infrastructure, such as schools, transportation systems, and parks; and social comparisons between individuals in different income groups, which may lead to stress and negative psychological reactions (Zimmerman and Bell 2006). Many of these factors might respond to programmatic (e.g., community development) or policy interventions. Neighborhood-level deprivation moderates the relationship between individual income inequality and mental health outcomes in that people living in poor areas suffer more mental health problems in the face of higher inequality (Zimmerman and Bell 2006). In one of the first longitudinal, nationally representative studies examining inequality and mental health, state-level income inequality was independently associated with depression rates among women but not men; therefore, gender may be a moderator (Pabayo et al. 2013). Finally, age and physical health have been shown to be moderators: among older adults, people with more physical ailments have worse mental health outcomes related to inequality (Zimmerman and Bell 2006). Although some of these moderators cannot be altered, they could still guide the targeting of public health interventions.

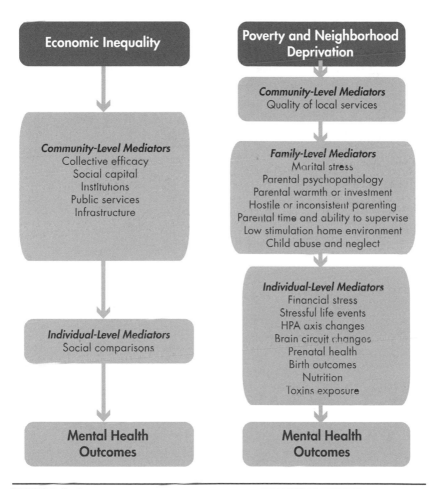

FIGURE 6–2.   Mediators of the links between economic social determinants and mental health.

HPA axis=hypothalamic-pituitary-adrenal axis.

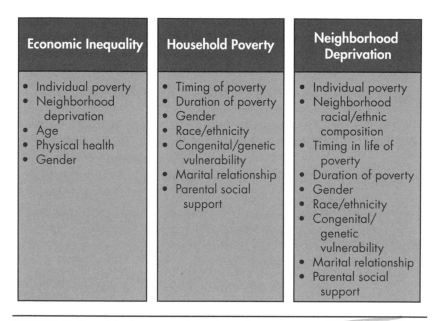

Economic Inequality	Household Poverty	Neighborhood Deprivation
• Individual poverty • Neighborhood deprivation • Age • Physical health • Gender	• Timing of poverty • Duration of poverty • Gender • Race/ethnicity • Congenital/genetic vulnerability • Marital relationship • Parental social support	• Individual poverty • Neighborhood racial/ethnic composition • Timing in life of poverty • Duration of poverty • Gender • Race/ethnicity • Congenital/genetic vulnerability • Marital relationship • Parental social support

FIGURE 6–3. Moderators of the links between economic social determinants and mental health.

Decades of work have shown unequivocally that poverty in childhood is toxic to mental health and cognitive outcomes. In numerous cross-sectional and longitudinal observational studies, childhood poverty has been associated with lower school achievement; worse cognitive, behavioral, and attention-related outcomes; higher rates of delinquency; and higher rates of depressive and anxiety disorders (McLoyd 1998; Yoshikawa et al. 2012). Childhood poverty is also associated with various negative social and mental health outcomes in adulthood, including lower academic achievement, arrests, posttraumatic stress disorder, and major depressive disorder (Nikulina et al. 2011).

In 2003, a groundbreaking study, the Great Smoky Mountains Study, was published about a serendipitous natural experiment that illuminated the relationship between childhood poverty and mental health (Costello et al. 2003). Between 1993 and 2000, the investigators followed a representative sample of 1,420 children in rural North Carolina as part of an epidemiological study involving annual psychiatric assessments. Children were between 9 and 13 years old at intake, and American Indians were oversampled. About halfway through the study, a casino opened, with a legal agreement to give every American Indian man, woman, and child an annual percentage of the proceeds, which was substantial and increased over time. Over the course of the study, 14% of families moved out of poverty (ex-poor), 53% remained poor (persistently poor), and 32% were never poor. Before the casino opened, overall psychiatric symptom scores for the persistently poor and the ex-poor children were equivalent but were significantly higher than the symptom scores for the never poor. After the casino opened, a significant decrease occurred in symptom scores for the ex-poor, which became equivalent to never poor symptom scores and significantly lower than persistently poor scores. No changes occurred in symptom scores for the persistently poor. Subanalyses found that changes in symptoms were almost entirely explained by behavioral (as opposed to emotional) symptoms and that these changes were mediated by changes in parents' abilities to provide adequate supervision. Further analyses showed that these results were explained by the ex-poor parents having fewer time constraints after the casino opened. The Great Smoky Mountains Study not only provides strong support for social causation but also reveals important leverage points for interventions designed to break the links between poverty and negative mental health outcomes, such as parental supervision ability and time constraints.

Although especially toxic in childhood, poverty is also detrimental to mental health during adulthood. In a large, nationally representative longitudinal study, lower household income was associated with suicide attempts and higher rates of almost every psychiatric disorder in adulthood, with the exception of obsessive-compulsive disorder (Sareen et al. 2011). As evidence for social causation, decreases in household income preceded and predicted the onset of mood, anxiety, and substance use disorders (Sareen et al. 2011). Poverty in adulthood has also been associated with psychological distress, depression, and completed suicide (Kingston 2013; Li et al. 2011). A recent, highly innovative report demonstrated that poverty depletes cognition (Mani et al. 2013), supporting both social causation (i.e., poverty was shown to affect cognition, not vice versa) and social selection (i.e., those whose cognition is affected by poverty may have diminished ability to transcend poverty). Specifically, stressful thoughts about finances lowered cognitive performance among poor but not among well-off experimental subjects in the United States.

Factors mediating the relationship between poverty and poor mental health have been identified at both the individual and family levels; many such factors are mutable and therefore present key opportunities for clinical and policy intervention. Individual-level mediators include financial stress, exposure to chronic and acute stressful life events, hypothalamic-pituitary-adrenal axis changes, brain circuit changes (in regions underpinning language processing and executive function), prenatal health and birth outcomes, nutrition, and toxin exposure (e.g., lead) (Hackman et al. 2010; McLoyd 1998; Yoshikawa et al. 2012). Family-level mediators include marital stress, parental psychopathology (especially depression), parental warmth or investment, hostile and/or inconsistent parenting, low-stimulation home environments, and child abuse and neglect (McLoyd 1998; Nikulina et al. 2011). The timing and duration of poverty moderate the relationships with mental health, in that poverty at a younger age and for longer is associated with worse outcomes (National Institute of Child Health and Human Development Early Child Care Research Network 2005). Although age is not mutable, this finding emphasizes the urgency of intervening when children are exposed to poverty at a young age in order to attempt to avoid the cumulative and durable damage that early poverty can exact over a lifetime. High-quality marital relationships and greater parental social support tend to mitigate the effects of poverty on mental health (McLoyd 1998), although recent research with poor, depressed mothers in Chicago suggested that these protective effects may, unfortunately, be more limited than previously thought (Kingston 2013). Although the identified moderators and quasi-experiments such as the Great Smoky Mountains Study provide strong evidence for the role of social causation in the link between poverty and mental health, some evidence also indicates that poverty leads to mental health and developmental problems that in turn prevent individuals and families from leaving poverty, creating an intergenerational vicious cycle between social causation and selection (McLoyd 1998).

Poverty that is geographically concentrated, often in urban areas, has been shown to be particularly detrimental to mental health, especially for children. High rates of unemployment, crime and criminal justice system involvement, adolescent delinquency, social and physical neighborhood disorder, single-parent households, and residential instability typically characterize poor neighborhoods (Chow et al. 2005). Neighborhood deprivation has been associated with many of the same mental health problems as household poverty, even after controlling for individual-level poverty, and has a particularly strong relationship to crime and juvenile delinquency (Chow et al. 2005; Chung and Steinberg 2006). Although the great majority of the literature on area-level deprivation has been conducted within urban neighborhoods, rural poverty has been linked to both anxiety and aggression in youth (Smokowski et al. 2013), as well as depression among women (Simmons et al. 2008). Institutional and structural mediators explaining the relationship between neighborhood deprivation and mental health outcomes include the quality of local services and schools; the physical state of the neighborhood, including infrastructure and green space; and the physical and social distance between residents (Chung and Steinberg 2006). Community-level mediators include collective efficacy (Sampson et al. 1997), socialization by adults, peer influences, social networks, exposure to crime and violence, and safety fears (Chung and Steinberg 2006). Individual-level poverty moderates the relationship between neighborhood deprivation and mental health, with poorer families being affected more adversely by area-level poverty (Chow et al. 2005).

The Moving to Opportunity study represented an ambitious social experiment designed to test the relationship between neighborhood deprivation and mental health. From 1994 to 1998, 4,604 low-income families living in public housing in New York City, Baltimore, Boston, Chicago, and Los Angeles were randomly assigned to three groups: 1) the low-poverty voucher (LPV) group received assistance to move to a census tract with a poverty rate of less than 10% and to remain there for at least a year, 2) the traditional voucher (TRV) group received vouchers to move with no restrictions, and 3) the control group received no assistance throughout the study period (Ludwig et al. 2012). The findings were mixed and controversial, with most initial analyses occurring only within separate sites. Some site-specific analyses showed improvements in educational attainment and psychological symptoms after 2–3 years for boys in the LPV and TRV groups, especially younger boys (Leventhal and Brooks-Gunn 2004). Educational attainment improvements seemed to disappear by 5 years, and school engagement and grades were actually worse for the LPV group than for control groups in some analyses (Leventhal et al. 2005). Adolescent girls in the LPV group had less psychological distress, anxiety, and substance use and were less likely to be arrested than adolescent girls in the control group. However, adolescent boys in the LPV group were not better off than adolescent boys in the control group, reported more substance use and behavioral problems, and were more likely to be arrested for property crimes than adolescent boys in the control group (Osypuk et al. 2012). Findings were most consistently positive for adults in the LPV group, who had significantly better physical and mental health and subjective well-being, even after 10–15 years (Ludwig et al. 2012). Although the overall findings provide support for a social causation relationship between neighborhood deprivation and negative mental health outcomes, they also signal the need for caution in designing interventions. For instance, it may be important to identify, optimize, and invest in strengths within impoverished communities rather than to characterize them in a simplified negative manner and thus encourage residents to abandon their communities (Jackson et al. 2009).

Poverty and Neighborhood Deprivation in the Clinical Setting

Case Example: How Individual and Neighborhood Poverty Affect Mental Health

Cynthia Clancy is a 40-year-old, single, unemployed African American woman living in public housing in one of the poorest neighborhoods of New York City. She currently lives with both a teenage son and an adult son in a two-bedroom apartment. Her adult son was diagnosed with attention-deficit/hyperactivity disorder as a child and has had legal troubles leading to periods of incarceration as an adult. Her adult daughter lives in a family shelter and frequently leaves her two young children at Ms. Clancy's apartment for extended periods of time. Ms. Clancy has a long history of depression, alcohol use disorder, and cannabis use disorder, all mostly untreated, and a medical history of hypertension, with poor primary care follow-up. She grew up in a single-mother household in the same neighborhood where she now lives and was sexually abused by her maternal uncle when she was 10 years old.

After a stressful argument with her adult son, Ms. Clancy presented to a clinic complaining of depressed mood, anhedonia, low energy, poor concentration, difficulty sleeping, decreased appetite, hopelessness, and passing thoughts of suicide without any intent or plan to harm herself. She also admitted to drinking between 6 and 12 beers per day and smoking a joint of marijuana every other day for the past several months, which represented a significant increase in her use of both substances. Although she reported mostly depressive symptoms, on mental status examination she presented as highly anxious, with some minor psychomotor agitation, rapid speech, circumstantial thinking when describing stressful situations at home, and repeated vague references to "stress" in her life. She frequently became tearful in the initial interview, especially when discussing family conflict. Although she was not able to recall details of previous mental health treatment, she thought that similar symptoms had responded to an antidepressant medication about 10 years ago.

Ms. Clancy was started on a selective serotonin reuptake inhibitor. She returned to the clinic 3 weeks later, reporting some improvement in depressive symptoms but with continued heavy alcohol use and frequent marijuana use. She was started on naltrexone, and the dosage of her antidepressant medication was increased. Two weeks later, she reported a reduction in her alcohol use and depressive symptoms, and it was assumed that she was on her way to recovery. However, 2 weeks later, Ms. Clancy returned to the clinic in crisis, reporting a return of all her depressive symptoms and an increase in both alcohol and marijuana use. On further questioning, she revealed that she was having great difficulty paying rent and was at risk of losing her apartment. Her daughter had also left her children with Ms. Clancy for the entire week, often staying overnight herself, creating a crowded, stressful environment in Ms. Clancy's home.

Ms. Clancy was referred to a local housing advocacy and community development organization to help manage her finances and avoid eviction and to provide problem-based support for the numerous stressors in her family's life. During the next several months, she missed several appointments, but when she did attend them, her symptoms were related much more closely to stressors in her life than to her medication dosage or adherence. When particularly stressful events occurred, she would present as frantically anxious, labile, circumstantial, and hopeless. One evening when her grandchildren and all three of her children were staying at her apartment, her daughter's ex-boyfriend broke down the door in search of her daughter and had a physical altercation with her adult son. During the altercation, Ms. Clancy developed chest pain, and her daughter called 911. On arrival at the emergency department, her blood pressure was noted to be 200/100, and she was admitted to the medical service.

Assessing and Addressing Poverty and Related Risk Factors in the Clinical Setting

Although it is always important for clinicians to assess the relationship between psychosocial factors and symptoms, it is particularly important in the context of poverty and neighborhood deprivation. As Ms. Clancy's case demonstrates, the contexts of poverty, neighborhood deprivation, and other social determinants of mental health can create a milieu of risk factors that combine to severely impair mental health. Although taking a detailed account of symptoms and treatment response remains vital, the economic social determinants of mental health often create so much stress that any expected illness course or treatment response is overwhelmed. Mental health providers can take a two-step approach to assess the impact of economic factors on mental health. First, they can assess, document, and attempt to address the mutable mediating and moderating factors shown in Figures 6–2 and 6–3. Second, they can assess the effects of poverty and neighborhood deprivation at the multiple levels of influence shown in Figure 6–1. This assessment involves asking not only about the individual patient but also about his or her household, family members, and neighborhood conditions.

Unfortunately, poverty is also associated with poor access to care, and clinicians in low-resource settings often face more time pressure than even the typical rushed mental health professional. In addition, like Ms. Clancy, economically disadvantaged patients tend to have chaotic and stressful lives that prevent them from following up with care in a way that would facilitate addressing their often complex clinical and social needs. Therefore, a careful evaluation of economic contributors to symptoms over time should be followed by appropriate referrals to organizations and programs able to address economic stressors. Sometimes such services can be integrated with clinical treatment, such as when job training or housing services are offered alongside psychiatric care in programs for individuals with serious mental illnesses. However, social services often carry the added advantage of being deliverable in nonclinical settings (e.g., home and schools), which are more convenient and potentially more comfortable for patients. Although the specific landscape of available services will depend on the local community, clinicians' awareness of and attention to the role of economic factors in mental health are the first vital step. Even if all a clinician does is pause to consider and discuss poverty-related risk factors before increasing a medication dosage or changing a diagnosis, the care provided will potentially improve through enhanced empathy for the patient, a better understanding of symptom etiology, and possibly avoiding unnecessary side effects. Going a step further, providers might consider helping their hospital or organization develop a local social services referral guide.

Even when such pragmatic steps are taken in an effort to make the most of available local resources, it is important to recognize that this approach may be woefully lacking in the face of systemic, pervasive inequality and economic deprivation for a host of reasons. First, in many impoverished communities, local services may be deficient or nonexistent. Second, even in relatively service-rich areas, generations of structural injustice may have damaged the social fabric of communities, strength of families, and resilience of individuals enough to make many services impotent. For instance, it is difficult to imagine a referral source that might remedy the destruction of social networks and wide-scale demoralization caused by the incarceration of two or three generations of men in many poor, mostly racial/ethnic minority neighborhoods in the United States. Third, because of entrenched bureaucracy and programmatic barriers such as rigid means testing or punitive sanctions, many programs can be either inaccessible or even harmful to those most in need of help. Finally, the experience of chronic poverty and neighborhood-level deprivation may cause so much stress in certain individuals and communities that it leads to a decreased ability or willingness to make use of available resources as a result of a deep-seated combination of distrust, exhaustion, and hopelessness that renders people less able to take advantage of well-meaning efforts to help. In a way, this perspective can be viewed as an understandable technique for coping with chronic stress and deprivation and may partially explain the perplexing interplay between social causation and social selection identified in some research. What can individual clinicians do in the face of such seemingly insurmountable barriers? The answer lies outside of clinics, hospitals, and traditional roles as health care providers treating patients and instead is found in communities, society as a whole, and roles as citizens advocating for policy and social change.

Policy Approaches to Inequality, Poverty, and Neighborhood Deprivation as Social Determinants of Mental Health

Referring again to Figure 6–1, it is clear that the most comprehensive approach to addressing the economic social determinants of mental health is to intervene on the multiple levels on which inequality and poverty have been shown to affect mental health outcomes. Although the efforts of individual clinicians can mitigate certain mediators and moderators linking poverty with mental illnesses on the individual and family levels, factors at the neighborhood, community, and societal levels can be addressed most effectively through policies and large-scale prevention-oriented programs.

Government-Supported Programs Affecting Poverty and Neighborhood Deprivation

Any program that provides support to individuals, families, and communities coping with the web of risk factors associated with poverty and neighborhood deprivation has the potential to improve mental health. Although myriad government-supported programs exist, a few examples are illustrative. Robust jobs programs have been shown to improve both economic and mental health outcomes over the long term (Vinokur et al. 2000). Community development and neighborhood organization programs also hold promise to improve community infrastructure, collective efficacy (Ohmer and Beck 2006), and safety. Given the particularly toxic effects of poverty on children's mental health and development, it is encouraging that early intervention–focused educational programs seem to be capable of conferring long-term benefits on functioning, improving childhood cognitive, educational, behavioral, and mental health outcomes (Reynolds et al. 2001). Although some effects tend to diminish, such as improvements in intelligence quotient (IQ), this finding may be largely due to control groups catching up in school. Other effects (e.g., school attainment, employment, income, and criminal justice involvement) have been shown to last for years and even decades (Reynolds et al. 2001, 2007). Intensive programs that start at a younger age are more effective, and public programs like Head Start have been shown to be both effective and cost-effective (Barnett 1998). Finally, cash transfer programs conditional on receipt of services such as prenatal care, pediatric primary care, and educational workshops have been shown to improve outcomes such as maternal depressive symptoms and child behavioral problems (Ozer et al. 2009, 2011).

Policies Breaking the Links Between Inequality, Poverty, and Poor Mental Health

Given the strong evidence for the role of social causation in the relationships between economic inequality, poverty, and poor mental health, addressing the economic social determinants of mental health directly would seem to be a way to greatly improve mental health on a population level. Ever since President Franklin D. Roosevelt's New Deal during the Great Depression, followed several decades later by President Lyndon B. Johnson's War on Poverty and Great Society initiatives, policy makers in the United States have been attempting in earnest, with varying and arguable measures of success, to alleviate inequality and eradicate poverty. Furthermore, although a general discussion of macroeconomic trends, labor market dynamics, and fiscal policy is beyond the scope of this chapter, it is clear that public policies still hold the greatest potential to affect the economic social determinants of mental health. From a public health perspective, policies that directly increase income for the poor and reduce societal inequality would broadly improve mental health. For instance, federal programs such as the Earned Income and Child and Dependent Care tax credits, Medicare, Medicaid, and Social Security have been quite effective in reducing poverty and its deleterious effects on health (Yoshikawa et al. 2012) and have, as a result, made the United States a more equal society. With this in mind, it is reasonable to assume that other economic initiatives that increase income and financial security, such as raising the minimum wage and a strong system of unemployment insurance, would also improve and protect mental health. Welfare or public assistance also represents a vital public commitment to preventing abject poverty, especially for the poor families with children most at risk of developing lifelong physical and mental health problems related to low income. However, recent analyses show that the Temporary Assistance for Needy Families (TANF) program currently provides far less real income to the nation's poorest families in most states than welfare programs did prior to reform legislation in 1996 (Floyd and Schott 2013). Given recent economic, political, and government budgetary challenges that have burdened the poor far more than the wealthy, more can and must be done through economic policy and social safety net programs to blunt mental health damage from the recently rising tide of concentrated poverty and inequality.

Promoting Better Economic Equality and Security: A Role for Everyone

In order to break the complex links between economic inequality, poverty, and poor mental health, mental health professionals and public health advocates need to take a multilevel, prevention-oriented approach. Diverse methods and skill sets are necessary to address the various levels represented in Figure 6–1. Although focusing on the top of the diagram holds the greatest potential for creating conditions for widespread improvements in mental health, policy change occurs in fits and starts and is often an exceedingly slow process with numerous setbacks. Therefore, although smaller in scale, improvements at the neighborhood, family, and individual levels through programmatic and clinical interventions are a vital part of the process. Through increased awareness and careful assessment of the economic social determinants of mental health, as well as clinical intervention and referral to social services programs, mental health professionals can help their patients avoid some of the negative consequences of inequality and poverty. Perhaps more importantly, clinicians can collectively use their political power and public trust as health care providers to advocate for policies and programmatic funding priorities that address inequality and poverty as social determinants of mental health. Both history and recent trends show just how difficult this can be. Although many are harmed by increasing inequality, there are relatively few powerful, vested interests that clearly benefit. Furthermore, political gridlock has recently reached an all-time high, putting a damper on policy solutions, particularly those involving public spending. However, against these odds, mental health professionals and public health advocates must attempt to draw attention to and alter the economic determinants of mental health on a broad scale. This advocacy likely represents the most potent way of improving the public's physical health and mental health and preventing psychiatric disability on a large scale.

Key Points

- Economic factors, including inequality, poverty, and neighborhood deprivation, are key social determinants of mental health. In the health literature, economic inequality is most often defined as income inequality, poverty using the federal poverty level, and neighborhood deprivation through an array of metrics. Economic inequality and poverty have been increasing in the United States for several decades, particularly among children—an unfortunate trend that has accelerated recently.

- The economic social determinants of mental health affect outcomes on multiple levels, including the societal, community, neighborhood, family, and individual levels. Therefore, a multilevel approach to addressing the relationships between economic factors and poor mental health and mental illnesses is most likely to be effective.

- To grasp the complex social epidemiology literature on the economic social determinants of health and mental health, it is important to understand the distinction between social causation and social selection, as well as the conceptual meaning of both mediating and moderating variables.

- Income inequality, poverty, and neighborhood deprivation have been linked to a wide array of negative mental health outcomes across the life span, with particularly deleterious and durable effects in children. Examining variables mediating and moderating the relationships between economic factors and mental health both increases understanding of these relationships and identifies opportunities to intervene.

- Although mental health providers have an important role in assessing and addressing the economic determinants of mental health at the clinical level, advocating for social and policy change at the community and societal levels represents the most potent way to improve the public's physical health and mental health.

References

Barnett WS: Long-term cognitive and academic effects of early childhood education on children in poverty. Prev Med 27(2):204–207, 1998 9578996

Boydell J, van Os J, McKenzie K, et al: The association of inequality with the incidence of schizophrenia—an ecological study. Soc Psychiatry Psychiatr Epidemiol 39(8):597–599, 2004 15300368

Chow JC, Johnson MA, Austin MJ: The status of low-income neighborhoods in the post-welfare reform environment: mapping the relationship between poverty and place. J Health Soc Policy 21(1):1–32, 2005 16418126

Chung HL, Steinberg L: Relations between neighborhood factors, parenting behaviors, peer deviance, and delinquency among serious juvenile offenders. Dev Psychol 42(2):319–331, 2006 16569170

Clark AM, DesMeules M, Luo W, et al: Socioeconomic status and cardiovascular disease: risks and implications for care. Nat Rev Cardiol 6(11):712–722, 2009 19770848

Costello EJ, Compton SN, Keeler G, et al: Relationships between poverty and psychopathology: a natural experiment. JAMA 290(15):2023–2029, 2003 14559956

DeNavas-Walt C, Proctor BD, Smith JC: Income, Poverty, and Health Insurance Coverage in the United States: 2012. Washington, DC, U.S. Census Bureau, 2013

Diez-Roux AV: Multilevel analysis in public health research. Annu Rev Public Health 21:171–192, 2000 10884951

Durkheim E: Suicide: A Study in Sociology (1897). Glencoe, IL, Free Press of Glencoe, 1951

Floyd I, Schott L: TANF Cash Benefits Continued to Lose Value in 2013. Washington, DC, Center on Budget Policy and Priorities, 2013

Frohlich KL, Corin E, Potvin L: A theoretical proposal for the relationship between context and disease. Sociol Health Illn 23(6):776–797, 2001

Gould E: The Top One Percent Take Home 20 Percent of America's Income. Washington, DC, Economic Policy Institute, July 18, 2013. Available at: http://www.epi.org/publication/top-1-earners-home-20-americas-income. Accessed July 20, 2013.

Hackman DA, Farah MJ, Meaney MJ: Socioeconomic status and the brain: mechanistic insights from human and animal research. Nat Rev Neurosci 11(9):651–659, 2010 20725096

Jackson L, Langille L, Lyons R, et al: Does moving from a high-poverty to lower-poverty neighborhood improve mental health? A realist review of "Moving to Opportunity". Health Place 15(4):961–970, 2009 19427806

Kingston S: Economic adversity and depressive symptoms in mothers: do marital status and perceived social support matter? Am J Community Psychol 52(3–4):359–366, 2013 24122088

Kondo N, Sembajwe G, Kawachi I, et al: Income inequality, mortality, and self rated health: meta-analysis of multilevel studies. BMJ 339:b4471, 2009 19903981

Krieger N, Waterman P, Chen JT, et al: Zip code caveat: bias due to spatiotemporal mismatches between zip codes and US census-defined geographic areas—the Public Health Disparities Geocoding Project. Am J Public Health 92(7):1100–1102, 2002 12084688

Leventhal T, Brooks-Gunn J: A randomized study of neighborhood effects on low-income children's educational outcomes. Dev Psychol 40(4):488–507, 2004 15238038

Leventhal T, Fauth RC, Brooks-Gunn J: Neighborhood poverty and public policy: a 5-year follow-up of children's educational outcomes in the New York City Moving to Opportunity demonstration. Dev Psychol 41(6):933–952, 2005 16351338

Li Z, Page A, Martin G, et al: Attributable risk of psychiatric and socio-economic factors for suicide from individual-level, population-based studies: a systematic review. Soc Sci Med 72(4):608–616, 2011 21211874

Ludwig J, Duncan GJ, Gennetian LA, et al: Neighborhood effects on the long-term well-being of low-income adults. Science 337(6101):1505–1510, 2012 22997331

Mani A, Mullainathan S, Shafir E, et al: Poverty impedes cognitive function. Science 341(6149):976–980, 2013 23990553

McLoyd VC: Socioeconomic disadvantage and child development. Am Psychol 53(2):185–204, 1998 9491747

Messias E, Eaton WW, Grooms AN: Economic grand rounds: income inequality and depression prevalence across the United States: an ecological study. Psychiatr Serv 62(7):710–712, 2011 21724781

Metcalfe A, Lail P, Ghali WA, et al: The association between neighbourhoods and adverse birth outcomes: a systematic review and meta-analysis of multi-level studies. Paediatr Perinat Epidemiol 25(3):236–245, 2011 21470263

Muramatsu N: County-level income inequality and depression among older Americans. Health Serv Res 38(6 Pt 2):1863–1883, 2003 14727801

Nandi A, Galea S, Ahern J, et al: What explains the association between neighborhood-level income inequality and the risk of fatal overdose in New York City? Soc Sci Med 63(3):662–674, 2006 16597478

National Institute of Child Health and Human Development Early Child Care Research Network: Duration and developmental timing of poverty and children's cognitive and social development from birth through third grade. Child Dev 76(4):795–810, 2005 16026497

Nikulina V, Widom CS, Czaja S: The role of childhood neglect and childhood poverty in predicting mental health, academic achievement and crime in adulthood. Am J Community Psychol 48(3–4):309–321, 2011 21116706

Ohmer M, Beck E: Citizen participation in neighborhood organizations in poor communities and its relationship to neighborhood and organizational collective efficacy. J Sociol Soc Welf 33(1):179–202, 2006

Organisation for Economic Co-operation and Development: OECD Factbook 2011–2012: Economic, Environmental, and Social Statistics. Paris, Organisation for Economic Co-operation and Development, 2012

Osypuk TL, Tchetgen EJ, Acevedo-Garcia D, et al: Differential mental health effects of neighborhood relocation among youth in vulnerable families: results from a randomized trial. Arch Gen Psychiatry 69(12):1284–1294, 2012 23045214

Ozer EJ, Fernald LC, Manley JG, et al: Effects of a conditional cash transfer program on children's behavior problems. Pediatrics 123(4):e630–e637, 2009 19336354

Ozer EJ, Fernald LC, Weber A, et al: Does alleviating poverty affect mothers' depressive symptoms? A quasi-experimental investigation of Mexico's Oportunidades programme. Int J Epidemiol 40(6):1565–1576, 2011 21737404

Pabayo R, Kawachi I, Gilman SE: Income inequality among American states and the incidence of major depression. J Epidemiol Community Health 68(2):110–115, 2014 24064745

Pickett KE, Wilkinson RG: Child wellbeing and income inequality in rich societies: ecological cross sectional study. BMJ 335(7629):1080–1086, 2007 18024483

Piketty T, Saez E: Income inequality in the United States, 1913–1998. Q J Econ 118:1–39, 2003

Reynolds AJ, Temple JA, Robertson DL, et al: Long-term effects of an early childhood intervention on educational achievement and juvenile arrest: a 15-year follow-up of low income children in public schools. JAMA 285(18):2339–2346, 2001 11343481

Reynolds AJ, Temple JA, Ou SR, et al: Effects of a school-based, early childhood intervention on adult health and well-being: a 19-year follow-up of low-income families. Arch Pediatr Adolesc Med 161(8):730–739, 2007 17679653

Sampson RJ, Raudenbush SW, Earls F: Neighborhoods and violent crime: a multilevel study of collective efficacy. Science 277(5328):918–924, 1997 9252316

Sareen J, Afifi TO, McMillan KA, et al: Relationship between household income and mental disorders: findings from a population-based longitudinal study. Arch Gen Psychiatry 68(4):419–427, 2011 21464366

Sen A: Development as Freedom. Oxford, UK, Oxford University Press, 1999

Simmons LA, Braun B, Charnigo R, et al: Depression and poverty among rural women: a relationship of social causation or social selection? J Rural Health 24(3):292–298, 2008 18643807

Smokowski PR, Cotter KL, Robertson CIB, et al: Anxiety and aggression in rural youth: baseline results from the rural adaptation project. Child Psychiatry Hum Dev 44(4):479–492, 2013 23108500

Syme SL: Historical perspective: the social determinants of disease—some roots of the movement. Epidemiol Perspect Innov 2(1):2, 2005 15840175

U.S. Department of Health and Human Services: Office of the Assistant Secretary for Planning and Evaluation: 2014 Poverty Guidelines. Washington, DC, U.S. Department of Health and Human Services, 2014. Available at: http://aspe.hhs.gov/poverty/14poverty.cfm. Accessed March 11, 2014.

Vinokur AD, Schul Y, Vuori J, et al: Two years after a job loss: long-term impact of the JOBS program on reemployment and mental health. J Occup Health Psychol 5(1):32–47, 2000 10658883

Wilkinson RG: Income distribution and life expectancy. BMJ 304(6820):165–168, 1992 1637372

World Health Organization: Preamble to the Constitution of the World Health Organization as adopted by the International Health Conference. New York, World Health Organization, 1948

Yoshikawa H, Aber JL, Beardslee WR: The effects of poverty on the mental, emotional, and behavioral health of children and youth: implications for prevention. Am Psychol 67(4):272–284, 2012 22583341

Zimmerman FJ, Bell JF: Income inequality and physical and mental health: testing associations consistent with proposed causal pathways. J Epidemiol Community Health 60(6):513–521, 2006 16698982

7

Food Insecurity

Michael T. Compton, M.D., M.P.H.

*There will never cease to be ferment in the world
unless people are sure of their food.*

Pearl S. Buck, 1892–1973

Being unsure of whether one will have enough food—as an individual, a family, or a community as a whole—is undoubtedly linked to anxiety, agitation, unrest, and poor mental health. Perhaps second only to air and water, food is the most essential of all human needs, yet most of us take for granted abundant food, good nutrition, and the absence of hunger. Food is not only a need; it is intimately linked to the mind and brain through its ability to immediately cease unpleasant sensations of hunger and because different types of food offer varying levels of reward. Furthermore, food is at the center of much of human culture and social experience. Thus, insufficient access to food is more encompassing than just nutritional insufficiency.

Far too many people in low- and middle-income countries—and even in developed, high-income countries, including the United States—are not sure they will have enough food to last through the month or the week (or are unsure where their food will come from or how they will get it). This uncertainty is known as *food insecurity*, defined as a condition in which the availability of nutritionally adequate and safe foods, or the ability to acquire such foods in socially acceptable

The author acknowledges the helpful feedback provided by Alisha Coleman-Jensen, Ph.D., David A. Pollack, M.D., and Kenneth S. Thompson, M.D.

145

ways, is limited or uncertain, most often because of constrained financial resources. Unfortunately, many Americans cannot afford or do not have ready access to enough nutritious foods. In addition to being anxiety provoking, food insecurity is a tremendous burden on one's capacity to thrive and succeed at anything in life or to even have an active mental life beyond the confines of securing food or facing the other related social challenges with which those who are hungry have to cope.

Food insecurity is a multidimensional construct involving deficiencies in quantity, quality, and access to nutritious and safe foods, which can be understood at both the societal level and the individual level (see Figure 7–1). The causes of food insecurity are complex, and its consequences are diverse and interrelated. For individuals, food insecurity is a socioenvironmental risk factor that is usually intertwined with other risk factors, such as poverty, unemployment, housing instability, violence and trauma, and limited education (poor education in general and poor health and food literacy in particular), as well as poor social support, social isolation, and loneliness.

Food insecurity affects not only the individual but also the community. Its impact on communities may compound other community-level risks, such as neighborhood disarray. At the societal level, food insecurity is a root cause of individual-level risk factors, linked to income inequality and neighborhood disenfranchisement. In a land of abundant food like the United States, the inability to access sufficient nutritious food reveals powerlessness, social exclusion, and unjust distribution of the most basic needs and opportunities. It also is evidence of market failure—a mismatch between demand and supply (i.e., insufficient demand due to insufficient money to buy) and thus an inability of the market to deliver a needed commodity. These circumstances have profound effects on individuals and communities alike.

This chapter explores the mental health consequences of food insecurity and presents both clinical and policy approaches to this social determinant of mental health. The anxiety-provoking uncertainty as to whether a person, household, or community will have enough nutritious food is a clinical, public health, and social justice problem of sufficient importance, even in the United States, to deserve heightened scrutiny. Despite the known link between food insecurity and poor mental health outcomes and mental illnesses, food insecurity is too often neglected by both clinicians (perhaps especially by mental health professionals) and policy makers. Although issues pertaining to overweight and obesity, corporate agriculture and the food industry, and dietary composition

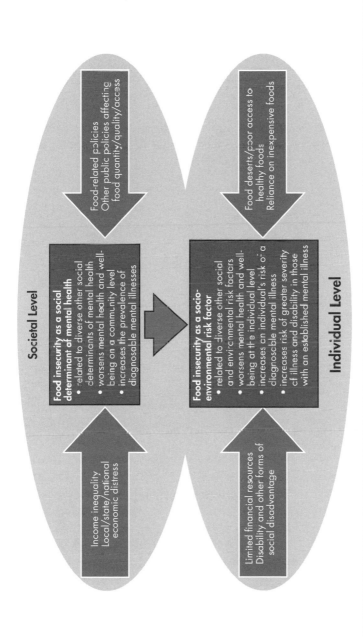

FIGURE 7–1. Food insecurity as a social determinant of mental health at the societal and individual levels.

are, to some extent, at the forefront of the modern American psyche (as exemplified by documentaries such as *Fast Food Nation, Food, Inc., Food Matters, Forks Over Knives, Fresh, Hungry for Change, Ingredients, Killer at Large, King Corn, Super Size Me, Vegucated,* and *The Weight of the Nation*), U.S. society gives less thought to food insecurity and its role in physical illnesses and social and mental distress (although the recent documentary *A Place at the Table* is a noteworthy exception).

Although the focus of this chapter is on food insecurity as a social determinant of mental health, many interesting and important food-related topics with implications for individual and community mental health are beyond this chapter's scope. To focus on food insecurity, we must unfortunately set aside topics that are certainly pertinent, such as the role of public education (and health and nutrition literacy in particular) in addressing dietary quality; the influence of advertising in shaping people's food choices; the mental health benefits of specific food components, such as mono- and polyunsaturated fatty acids and other "brain foods"; maternal and infant mental health benefits of breastfeeding; parenting skills pertaining to instilling healthy food preferences in children; the mental health impacts of eating together in social settings; and the mental health benefits of gardening and growing one's own food.

Food Insecurity: An Overview

Food security, food insecurity, and hunger are defined in Table 7–1. Food security is one of several conditions necessary for a population to be physically and mentally healthy and well nourished (Coleman-Jensen et al. 2012). Because health is a state of physical, emotional, behavioral, and social well-being and not merely the absence of disease, food security is, by definition, a social determinant of both physical health and mental health.

Prevalence of Food Insecurity in the United States

Food insecurity is a major problem affecting low-income countries and famine areas, leading to hunger, nutritional deficiencies, malnutrition, medical and social problems, and excesses in morbidity and mortality. However, food insecurity also occurs in high-income countries, including the United States. Since 1995, to supplement the nationally representative Current Population Survey of the U.S. Census Bureau, the U.S. Department of Agriculture (USDA) has conducted annual surveys on

TABLE 7–1. Definitions of food security, food insecurity, and hunger

	Definition	Reference
Food security	Exists "when all people at all times have access to sufficient, safe, nutritious food to maintain a healthy and active life." The concept of food security is commonly defined as including both physical and economic access to food that meets people's dietary needs as well as their food preferences.	World Food Summit of 1996 (World Health Organization 2014)
Food insecurity	Occurs "when there is uncertainty about future food availability and access, insufficiency in the amount and kind of food required for a healthy lifestyle, or the need to use socially unacceptable ways to acquire food" because of resource or physical constraint.	National Research Council (Wunderlich and Norwood 2006)
Hunger	Is "the uneasy or painful sensation caused by a lack of food...the recurrent and involuntary lack of access to food." Hunger may produce malnutrition over time and is a potential, although not necessary, consequence of food insecurity.	Expert working group of the American Institute of Nutrition (Anderson 1990)

food access and adequacy, food spending, and sources of food assistance for the U.S. population. Examples of food insecurity survey questions are shown in Table 7–2. Such survey items can be summed to derive useful cut points for defining levels of food security or insecurity; for example, *low food security* indicates reduced quality, variety, or desirability of diet but little or no indication of reduced food intake, whereas *very low food security* refers to multiple indications of disrupted eating patterns and reduced food intake.

In 2011, 17.9 million U.S. households (14.9%) were food insecure at some time during the year, and 6.8 million households (5.7%) had *very low* food security (Coleman-Jensen et al. 2012). Because the impact of food insecurity may be most profound when it occurs in childhood, it is particularly noteworthy that 20.6% of all U.S. households with children were food insecure at some time during the year, and although adults commonly shield children from the effects of household food insecurity by diverting food to them, in about half of these households, the children themselves were food insecure.

The prevalence of food insecurity varies substantially across the United States. Using combined data from 2009–2011 (allowing for more stable estimates), the USDA documents that some states have rates of household food insecurity of less than 10% (e.g., North Dakota, 7.8%; Virginia, 9.1%; New Hampshire, 9.6%), whereas others have rates in excess of 18% (e.g., Texas, 18.5%; Arkansas, 19.2%; Mississippi, 19.2%) (Coleman-Jensen et al. 2012). Between-state variations in the prevalence of food insecurity are driven by differences in states' populations (e.g., pertaining to education and employment) and differences in tax policies and the nature of participation in federal food and nutrition assistance programs. It is also noteworthy that the states with the highest rates of food insecurity tend to correspond to the states with the greatest degree of income inequality among their citizens, consistent with the observation across nations that a more equal distribution of resources equates to fewer people with food insecurity (Wilkinson and Pickett 2009).

In addition to state-to-state variation, the prevalence of food insecurity varies across demographic groups or circumstances. Rates of food insecurity are substantially higher than the national average in African American and Hispanic families, in households with incomes near or below the federal poverty level, in households with children (especially households headed by a single mother), and in large cities or in rural areas compared with those in suburban areas. Furthermore, food insecurity is much more prevalent in households with a working-age adult with a disability, including a mental health disability (Coleman-Jensen

---

TABLE 7–2. Examples of questions from the U.S. Adult Food
Security Survey

In the last 12 months:

Did you or other adults in your household ever cut the size of your
meals or skip meals because there wasn't enough money for food?

Did you ever eat less than you felt you should because there wasn't
enough money for food?

Were you ever hungry but didn't eat because there wasn't enough
money for food?

Did you lose weight because there wasn't enough money for food?

Did you or other adults in your household ever not eat for a whole day
because there wasn't enough money for food?

Source. Bickel et al. 2000

---

and Nord 2013). Many such households face other risks for poor mental
health (e.g., housing instability), again reinforcing the fact that such social risks tend to cluster together among the most socially and economically disadvantaged individuals, families, and communities. Recent
attention to *food deserts,* or areas characterized by poor access to healthy
and affordable foods, emphasizes that community-level social and spatial disparities in food access and dietary quality likely contribute to
health inequities (Walker et al. 2010). Modern methods for measuring
the food environment (e.g., geospatial analysis) hold promise for identifying community-level predictors of individual dietary quality and for
informing policy pertaining to the food environment.

Food Insecurity as a Social Determinant of Health

Diet is one of the principal determinants of many common health conditions, including the most prevalent chronic diseases affecting developed countries, such as cardiovascular disease, type 2 diabetes, and
cancer (Robertson et al. 2006). Food insecurity is associated with poorer
self-reported health status (Stuff et al. 2004), which is linked to many adverse health outcomes, and also with objectively measured health indicators such as hypertension and diabetes (Seligman et al. 2010). Food
insecurity may also be associated with increased inflammatory responses (Gowda et al. 2012), which in turn are tied to diverse morbidities, including cardiovascular diseases. Food insecurity is related not only to
incidence of many chronic diseases but also to the course of those dis-

eases; for example, food insecurity is predictive of poorer glycemic control among those with diabetes, partly driven by emotional distress and difficulty following a healthy diet (Seligman et al. 2012). Even short but repeated periods of food insecurity and hunger can have a cumulative adverse effect on health (Kirkpatrick et al. 2010).

One reason for the connection with chronic diseases is that food insecurity is complexly related to dietary quality. Individuals and families in the United States with constrained financial resources tend to spend more of their limited money on energy-dense but nutritionally barren foods that are high in refined sugars, saturated fats, and salt, as well as sugary drinks. Overreliance on processed foods and fast food—and resultant reduced dietary variety, low consumption of fresh fruits and vegetables, and insufficient intake of micronutrients such as the B complex vitamins—is associated with chronic diseases that are the leading causes of death in the United States. Thus, although food insecurity can cause hunger and reduced food intake, in the United States and other high-income countries where certain kinds of foods are generally available beyond the population's needs but others are not (which is a market failure, as noted above), food insecurity is paradoxically associated with overweight and obesity (Dinour et al. 2007; Institute of Medicine 2011; Larson and Story 2011).

Food insecurity has profound effects on the health of children. Sufficient and nutritious food is a requirement for optimal physical, cognitive, social, and emotional growth and development (Stang et al. 2006). Children from food-insecure households have a higher prevalence of many illnesses and higher hospitalization rates (Cook et al. 2004). Affected children are at increased risk for iron deficiency anemia, developmental delays, stunted growth, compromised immune function and infections, impaired attainment of social skills, learning delays, poor school performance, and behavioral and emotional problems.

Food Insecurity as a Social Determinant of Mental Health

There can be little doubt that food insecurity leads to psychological stress—anxiety, frustration, a sense of powerlessness, and disconnection from others. In terms of mental illnesses, food insecurity is most clearly linked to depressive disorders (Alaimo et al. 2002; Huddleston-Casas et al. 2009; Lent et al. 2009; Siefert et al. 2001; Whitaker et al. 2006). More limited research shows that it is also associated with other adverse mental health outcomes such as poor self-reported mental health status (Stuff et al. 2004) and generalized anxiety disorder (Whitaker et al. 2006).

The ways in which food insecurity affect mental health are complex. As Figure 7–2 shows, food insecurity (and hunger, when it is also present) undoubtedly leads to psychological stress, which triggers diverse physiological stress responses that elevate risk for mental illnesses such as depressive and anxiety disorders. Nutritional deficiencies have also been implicated in the etiology of depressive disorders and are likely risk factors for other mental illnesses. In addition to the effects of nutritional deficiencies on the incidence of diagnosable mental illnesses, even mild vitamin deficiencies can adversely affect mental health (e.g., increased irritability, nervousness, and poorer cognitive performance) (Heseker et al. 1992).

The effects of food insecurity on the mental health of children are even more profound than its effects on adults. Food insecurity affects academic performance, social skills, and other early markers of later risk for poor mental health and mental illnesses (Alaimo et al. 2001). Eating breakfast is important to cognitive functioning in children, and the negative cognitive and academic effects of skipping breakfast are even more apparent in children whose nutritional status is compromised (Hoyland et al. 2009). Children living in food-insecure households are at increased risk for symptoms of depression and anxiety, hyperactivity and inattention, and behavioral problems (Whitaker et al. 2006). Food insecurity among parents (and consequent stress, depression, and anxiety) adversely affects parenting practices (Zaslow et al. 2009), which, in turn, has negative impacts on physical and mental health outcomes of children (Bronte-Tinkew et al. 2007). As such, food insecurity likely has a transgenerational effect on mental health (and potentially even a transgenerational epigenetic effect given that nutrients and nutritional deficiencies can modify gene expression through epigenetic mechanisms). Furthermore, food insecurity itself, often embedded within an array of other socioeconomic disadvantages, can be, in effect, passed from one generation to the next.

Figure 7–2 indicates the link between food insecurity and overweight and obesity, which is mediated by a reliance on inexpensive, energy-dense foods (given that the cheapest calories one can buy in the United States are processed, junk, and fast foods). In childhood and adolescence, overweight and obesity are complexly related to academic and social outcomes (Sabia 2007), and in adulthood, overweight and obesity appear to be associated in some way with some mental illnesses, including mood disorders and schizophrenia (Compton et al. 2006; McElroy

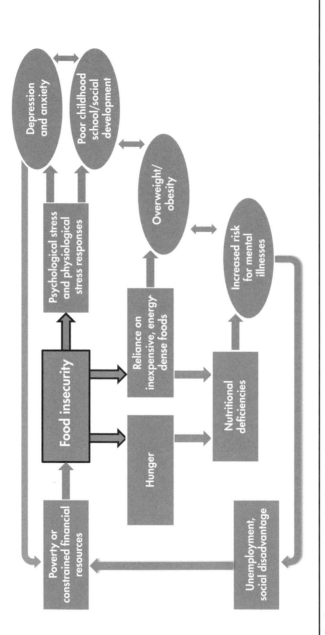

FIGURE 7–2. Some of the likely links between food insecurity and poor mental health.

et al. 2004). In light of the U.S. overweight and obesity epidemic, the burden of disease associated with the most prevalent mental illnesses, and the elevated morbidity and mortality associated with serious mental illnesses, concerted efforts are needed to better understand and address the links between food insecurity, overweight and obesity, and diverse mental illnesses across the life span.

Surprisingly little information is available on the causes and consequences of food insecurity among persons with serious mental illnesses such as psychotic disorders. Individuals with serious mental illnesses are at especially high risk of being socially and economically disadvantaged and are likely at particularly high risk for food insecurity because these disorders often impede gainful employment, greatly limiting financial resources. The particular social circumstances that plague persons with serious mental illnesses (e.g., high rates of adverse life experiences, victimization, homelessness, and substance abuse in addition to joblessness and poverty) undoubtedly drive high rates of food insecurity and limit the effectiveness of food assistance programs. Like financially constrained persons without serious mental illnesses, this vulnerable population is likely to get caught in a cycle in which nutrition support benefits (if received) are spent within the first few days of the month, resulting in food insufficiency by the end of the month, forcing the person to revert to inexpensive, energy-dense junk and fast foods. Furthermore, for a variety of reasons, this population tends not to prepare fresh food and tends to eat alone.

Clearly, the relationship between food insecurity and poor mental health outcomes is complex. Although our focus has been on food insecurity as a social determinant of mental health, we must also consider mental health as a determinant of food insecurity. That is, bidirectional associations must be considered (Huddleston-Casas et al. 2009; Lent et al. 2009), such that food insecurity leads to poor mental health outcomes and poor mental health or mental illnesses exacerbate the underlying causes of food insecurity. Like having a disability more broadly (Coleman-Jensen and Nord 2013), having a serious mental illness is undoubtedly an important determinant of food insecurity. This association is likely mediated by specific symptoms (e.g., the negative symptoms of schizophrenia, neurocognitive deficits, and comorbid depression and anxiety) and impairments in psychosocial functioning (e.g., poor social networks and limited transportation), as well as society's stance toward those living with serious mental illnesses (e.g., stigma and social exclusion).

Food Insecurity and Food-Related Risk Factors in the Clinical Setting

As noted previously in the opening paragraphs of this chapter, food insecurity affects individuals, families, communities, and society at large. The social determinants of mental health must be addressed at the individual level (in the clinical setting), at the family level (through social services and local programs), and at the community and societal level (through local, state, and federal policy initiatives).

Case Example: Food Insecurity in the Context of a Serious Mental Illness

Dr. Lenora Jones is a family medicine physician employed by a federally qualified health center, working with a team of health professionals to help patients manage chronic conditions. She provides care primarily for Medicare beneficiaries, including Mai Breedlove, a 72-year-old woman with hypertension, diabetes, and hypercholesterolemia. At a routine visit, Mrs. Breedlove brings her 22-year-old granddaughter, Doba Breedlove, to the clinic for a mental health evaluation. Mrs. Breedlove reports that in the past 4 months, Doba lost her job, became isolated at home in her apartment, lost at least 20 pounds, and stopped paying her utility bills (causing electricity service to be discontinued); the day before, she lost her car because of repossession.

On conducting a brief mental status examination, Dr. Jones observes that Doba is guarded, suspicious, timid, and reluctant to give details about recent events. Doba softly mentions that people at her former job had been "electronically tracking" her and that recently, her apartment neighbors had become "accomplices" who make threatening comments that she hears through the vents in her apartment. Dr. Jones empathizes with the stress and fear that Doba must be experiencing and walks her down the hall to consult with Dr. Kyle Stevens, a psychiatrist who works in the clinic as an on-site mental health consultant. While Dr. Stevens meets with Doba to initiate an outpatient evaluation and treatment plan, Mrs. Breedlove expresses worry that although she will be able to temporarily pay Doba's rent, paying for her mental health care, utilities, and transportation will be difficult because of Mrs. Breedlove's own limited financial resources.

Dr. Jones, Dr. Stevens, and the broader health care team clearly have a complex case before them. Doba has signs and symptoms that appear to be consistent with an emerging psychotic disorder, complicated by major psychosocial stressors. Her psychosocial circumstances clearly must be addressed during the initial evaluation and treatment of what are likely positive and negative symptoms of a psychotic disorder. Preoccupied with standard, pressing aspects of the evaluation (e.g., ruling out a medical condition that might underlie the recent onset of symptoms, assessing for substance use, initiating treatment and the monitoring of response and side effects), her health care team might be accustomed to assigning lower priority to assessing and addressing potential social and environmental risk factors that could exacerbate Doba's illness or attenuate the effects of newly prescribed pharmacological and psychosocial treatments.

Among the social and environmental risks that can be considered are those pertaining to food and nutrition. What is the cause of Doba's recent weight loss? What is her diet like? Does Doba have food at home? Is she able to get to the grocery store and buy groceries? What is her current nutritional status? Might she have nutritional deficiencies comorbid with or complicating her recent-onset mental illness? How might food insecurity serve as a stressor or exacerbating factor as she embarks on a path toward recovery? Will prescribed psychotropic medications increase her appetite, and if so, how will that side effect interact with poor availability of healthy foods to accentuate weight gain? These questions, although obviously relevant to Doba's mental and psychosocial condition, are often missing from the psychiatric evaluation. The potential for hunger, the likelihood of poor dietary quality, and the possibility of nutritional deficiencies could all be considered part of the treatment plan.

Assessing Food Insecurity and Related Risk Factors in the Clinical Setting

Health care teams can routinely use a set of brief, standardized questions to screen for food insecurity. Although questionnaires used in national surveys of food insecurity typically take only a few minutes to administer, even more abbreviated versions have been developed for the screening of food insecurity in clinical settings. Examples of two-item (Hager et al. 2010) and even one-item (Kleinman et al. 2007) screening questions, preliminarily studied in clinical settings, are given in Table 7–3. These questions screen only for food insecurity; other screening is required for dietary quality. Screening can be performed by non-physician health care team members, or screening questions can be added to intake surveys completed by patients or caregivers before the clinical encounter. For patients screening affirmatively, additional assessment of possible food insecurity is required.

How Clinicians Can Address Food Insecurity and Related Risk Factors

The crucial initial step in addressing food insecurity in the clinical setting is to begin routinely asking about it, which need not add excessive time to the typical clinical encounter. Addressing food insecurity (and,

TABLE 7–3. Examples of two- and one-item food insecurity screening questions for clinical settings

Hager et al. 2010	1. Within the past 12 months we worried whether our food would run out before we got money to buy more. ❑ Never true ❑ Sometimes true ❑ Often true 2. Within the past 12 months the food we bought just didn't last and we didn't have money to get more. ❑ Never true ❑ Sometimes true ❑ Often true
Kleinman et al. 2007	In the past month, was there any day when you or anyone in your family went hungry because you did not have enough money for food? ❑ Yes ❑ No

similarly, hunger, poor dietary quality, and nutritional deficiencies) can be thought of as comprising four key elements.

First, if a food-related risk factor is detected through screening, a more extensive evaluation is warranted. This evaluation entails determining the underlying causes; for example, is food insecurity stemming from restricted financial resources alone, or do limited transportation, insufficient local availability (e.g., food deserts), or psychiatric symptoms (e.g., negative symptoms of schizophrenia, depressive symptoms, anxiety symptoms associated with agoraphobia) create barriers? Second, because food insecurity is commonly experienced as a household risk, rather than solely an individual risk, family involvement in assessing and intervening on food insecurity is essential. Third, addressing food insecurity (which might partly begin to attend to poor dietary quality and any nutritional deficiencies also present in the context of food insecurity) requires familiarity with local food bank resources. Becoming acquainted with local resources is easy and at the health care team's fingertips, given extensive information and resources available online. For example, Feeding America's Web site (www.feedingamerica.org) has a food bank locator that identifies local resources in every state. Finally, the health care team can become more familiar with federal food and nutrition assistance programs (the administration of which varies somewhat across states), such as the Supplemental Nutrition Assistance Program (SNAP, formerly called the Food Stamp Program) and Special

Supplemental Nutrition Program for Women, Infants, and Children (WIC). Food-insecure families underuse available assistance programs (Kleinman et al. 2007), although families referred to such programs by health care providers are more likely to contact the recommended agencies and find them beneficial (Fleegler et al. 2007).

Assessing and ameliorating food insecurity among adults with mental illnesses will have favorable mental health effects for the entire family as well. Although many mental health professionals might not feel comfortable stepping into the role of nutritional consultant, dieticians or nutritionists in team-based practice settings can help patients plan meals that are inexpensive yet nutritious. Even if a nutritionist or dietary counselor is not routinely available, dietary counseling need not be burdensome during the standard clinical encounter. Federally produced dietary guidance, such as the *Dietary Guidelines for Americans* (U.S. Department of Agriculture and U.S. Department of Health and Human Services 2010), can help health professionals in their dietary counseling.

Because mental health clinicians might not be accustomed to asking about food insecurity and dietary quality when assessing other socioenvironmental risks, additional training would be beneficial. Models have been developed to train pediatric residents to screen for psychosocial risk factors, including food insecurity (Burkhardt et al. 2012; Feigelman et al. 2011), but routine monitoring of food insecurity is underused by health care professionals (Hoisington et al. 2012). Furthermore, training in this area is largely missing in psychiatry residencies and other training programs for mental health professionals.

In addition to assessing food-related social determinants of mental health in the clinical setting, truly addressing the problem of food insecurity will require primary care physicians, psychiatrists and other mental health professionals, and other clinicians to step outside of traditional professional boundaries to influence social welfare and economic policy initiatives (Siefert et al. 2001). Indeed, the American Medical Association's *Declaration of Professional Responsibility* encourages physicians to "advocate for social, economic, educational, and political changes that ameliorate suffering and contribute to human well-being." Such pronouncements that physicians and other health professionals have broader social and political responsibilities are not new; it was acknowledged well over 100 years ago that "medicine is a social science, and politics is nothing else but medicine on a large scale" and "if medicine is really to accomplish its great task, it must intervene in political and social life." (Both statements are attributed to German pathologist and anthropologist Rudolf Virchow.)

Policy Approaches to Food Insecurity as a Social Determinant of Mental Health

Politicians and policy makers have more potent influence over a society's physical and mental health than doctors in clinical settings. Although policy solutions to food insecurity are more powerful for the overall population than individual-level interventions delivered in the clinic, health care providers (including mental health professionals) often have limited training and confidence in their ability to influence policy. But clinicians, along with public health and policy professionals, have a role, if not a duty, in learning about and taking part in policy approaches to address the underlying causes of poor physical and mental health.

Local and State Programs Affecting Food Access and Dietary Quality

Households with limited resources employ a variety of methods to help meet their food needs; some participate in one or more of the federal food and nutrition assistance programs or obtain food from emergency food providers in their communities to supplement the food they can purchase (Coleman-Jensen et al. 2012). Initiatives by religious, volunteer, and community organizations and food banks to help those with constrained financial resources clearly have a role at the local level (Robertson et al. 2006). Clinicians who work with patient populations at risk for food insecurity can become more familiar with these local food banks, which can then be referred to as resources for patients and families.

Clinicians can also take part in local policy advocacy and programs that will affect food availability, access, and quality. Local interventions are effective, such as programs designed to increase availability of produce in small food stores in low-income neighborhoods with a high proportion of racial/ethnic minorities with limited access to healthy foods (Gittelsohn et al. 2012; Glanz and Yaroch 2004). For example, Gittelsohn and colleagues (2010) implemented an intervention trial called Baltimore Healthy Stores in nine food stores (two supermarkets and seven corner stores) in low-income, predominantly African American neighborhoods of Baltimore, with a comparison group of eight stores in other low-income neighborhoods in the city. The intervention included an environmental component to increase stocks of more nutritious foods and provided point-of-purchase promotions, including signage for healthy choices and interactive nutrition education sessions. These interventions significantly increased availability and sales of healthy foods and improved consumer knowledge and dietary behaviors (Gittelsohn et al. 2012). In addition to research interventions, local governments can consider ordinances pertaining to food retailer licensing (similar to tobacco retailer licensing laws) that would improve the local food environment, especially in low-income areas with poor access to healthy foods and an oversaturation of unhealthy foods (McLaughlin and Kramer 2012). Clinicians can have an influential voice in advocacy for such programs at the local level. Those interested in edible gardening, the movement around eating locally grown foods, and improvements in the food chain can also promote community development through community gardens and urban farms and can advance horticulture as a therapeutic or mental health promotion activity.

State-level policy approaches also have robust effects. For example, in 2004, the Pennsylvania Fresh Food Financing Initiative pioneered a statewide program that offered grants and loans to supermarket developers to build stores in underserved communities. The program made it easier for an estimated 500,000 residents to find healthier food in their communities (Giang et al. 2008). Many other state-level policies can influence food consumption and improve dietary quality (Hood et al. 2012); for example, in Michigan's Double Up Food Bucks program, if a SNAP recipient uses a SNAP card to buy food at a farmers' market, the amount of money spent is matched with up to $20 in tokens per day that can be used to buy Michigan-grown fruits and vegetables. Other pertinent programs and initiatives include farm-to-school programs (which allow local farmers to be suppliers of foods to schools), elimination of junk foods in vending machines in schools and health facilities, and food literacy initiatives (including school vegetable gardens) in early childhood and grade school.

Federal Policy and Programs Affecting Food Insecurity

About one in every four Americans participates in at least one of the 15 USDA domestic food and nutrition assistance programs (e.g., SNAP, WIC, the Child and Adult Care Food Program, the National School Lunch Program, and the School Breakfast Program), which together provide a nutritional safety net for millions of children and low-income adults (Oliveira 2012). These federal food and nutrition assistance programs represent a significant federal investment, accounting for more than two-thirds of USDA's budget. These programs appear to be effective at improving mental health; for example, studies of school breakfast programs suggest that they positively affect academic performance (which, in turn, is linked to better mental health outcomes), which is likely explained by improved nutrition, reduced sensations of hunger, greater energy and attention, and increased school attendance (Hoyland et al. 2009). However, only 57% of food-insecure households in the most recent national food security survey reported having participated in one or more of the three largest federal food and nutrition assistance programs in the previous month (Coleman-Jensen et al. 2012).

SNAP is highly successful at reducing rates of food insecurity in the United States, and to the extent that the program can be coupled with nutrition education, it might also prevent the development of diet-sensitive chronic diseases (Seligman et al. 2010). However, the average monthly SNAP benefit in 2011 was only $133.85 per beneficiary. Nearly half of SNAP's beneficiaries are children. Receiving SNAP benefits is often temporary, with half of all new participants leaving the program within 9 months. By design, the number of SNAP recipients typically rises during recessionary periods when unemployment rates rise and falls during periods of economic growth when those rates decline. Given the links between food insecurity and poorer physical and mental health outcomes, participation in SNAP and other federal food and nutrition assistance programs likely benefits the overall mental health of individuals, families, and the population. However, the specific mental health impacts of participating in such programs (including potentially negative impacts and stigmatization in addition to ostensible benefits) require further study.

Receiving federal food and nutrition assistance does not ensure consumption of nutritionally healthy food. Biologically distinct types of food that are intrinsically rich in micronutrients are necessary to support a nutritious diet. Some households participating in SNAP use a considerable portion of their benefits on unhealthy (but inexpensive) foods, such as sugar-sweetened beverages and processed foods. It has been suggested that SNAP's lack of focus on food quality might simultaneously exacerbate hunger and promote obesity (Ludwig et al. 2012) because energy-dense, nutritionally barren foods are often purchased with SNAP benefits. However, Gregory and colleagues (2013) recently found modest positive effects on diet among SNAP participants, primarily in the form of increasing consumption of whole fruit. Changes to SNAP are complex and require intensive scientific, ethical, financial, and public health analysis before being enacted (Laraia 2012). Food-related policy changes are also politically complex in light of the clear influence of agribusinesses and the processed food industry on food policies (Nestle 2002). Other programs have been modified, exemplified by the Healthy, Hunger-Free Kids Act of 2010, which required the National School Lunch Program, School Breakfast Program, and Child and Adult Care Food Program to improve nutritional quality (Ludwig et al. 2012).

Modifications to federal programs could improve the food environment more broadly, beyond effects for beneficiaries. As one example, the 2009 alignment of the WIC food package with the federal dietary guidelines added a monthly cash voucher of $6–$10 per participant to purchase fruits and vegetables. Although the primary policy aim was to improve WIC participants' dietary quality, a secondary effect was that community-level availability of fruits and vegetables increased because WIC-authorized vendors had to begin carrying fruits and vegetables in addition to processed and packaged foods (Havens et al. 2012; Zenk et al. 2012). This policy change, primarily aimed at WIC recipients, was associated with improvements in access to fruits and vegetables for the broader community, which is an important secondary outcome because rural, low-income, and predominantly minority neighborhoods have less access to healthy fruits and vegetables (Larson et al. 2009; Zenk et al. 2012).

Federal-level policy improvements could also address what are thought by many to be distorted and counterproductive food subsidy policies that support monoculture crops like corn and soybeans (used largely in processed food products) while minimally supporting fruit and vegetable production, which leads to artificially lower prices for the former and prohibitively higher prices for the latter. In addition to policies pertaining to the food and nutrition assistance programs, food insecurity can be reduced through more general public policy programs such as increasing the minimum wage. Even if a population's food supply is optimized in terms of nutritional goals, wide variation in diet and nutrition within the population will continue until poverty, income inequality, and pricing policies are addressed. Even then, persistence of poor dietary quality is likely, given cultural preferences and individual tastes. The latter suggests an ongoing role for public education in addition to policy measures.

Promoting the Availability of Adequate and Nutritious Foods: A Role for Everyone

Supporting good nutrition (healthy food in terms of both quantity and quality) across the life span from infancy to old age will improve the mental health of individuals, families, and communities and reduce the risk of mental illnesses. Although the particularly detrimental impact of food insecurity in childhood and adolescence has been emphasized in this chapter, many older adults are at risk for food insecurity and hunger (and thus malnutrition, which exacerbates chronic and acute health conditions), in part because of limited incomes, impaired mobility, and poor health (Wolfe et al. 1998). In addition to a focus on food security and nutrition across the life span, special attention is needed for vulnerable groups such as racial and ethnic minorities and those who are homeless or marginally housed. Although clinical- and policy-level interventions to prevent and ameliorate food insecurity across the life span could help reduce the incidence and prevalence of mental illnesses such as major depressive disorder (Heflin et al. 2005), researchers, the private and corporate sector, and citizens at large also have a role.

Regarding research, more work is needed on the exact nature of the role of food insecurity in causing and exacerbating specific mental illnesses and poor mental health more generally. Food insecurity, poor dietary quality, and nutritional deficiencies are among the least studied risk factors for poor mental health and mental illnesses. More research is also needed on how and the extent to which mental illnesses lead to food insecurity. Although perhaps somewhat tangential to the focus on food insecurity per se, many other topics pertinent to food-related social determinants of mental health at the community and societal levels deserve study. For example, are there differential mental health impacts (for farmers, local citizens, and consumers) of horticultural (plant-based) land use as opposed to animal-based agricultural land use? And are there differential mental health impacts of monoculture and monocropping practices of industrial agriculture versus diverse cropping, local foods, biodiversity, and heirloom gardening? Are there mental health impacts of programs supporting sustainable and participatory community agriculture (i.e., building community by growing food together)? Similarly, what are the mental health and recovery-related benefits of gardening as a psychosocial rehabilitation activity (and incorporating food-related psychoeducational activities) for persons receiving mental health services?

The duty to act to eliminate food insecurity does not fall on only clinicians, public health officials, policy makers, and researchers; the private sector and corporate America could have a powerful influence on improving access to healthy foods. Like most other social justice issues, each citizen can play a role, through advocacy, well-informed voting, and local community participation. Furthermore, adopting a human rights framework (i.e., actively engaging those affected in a right-to-food approach) has been suggested (Chilton and Rose 2009). As conveyed in the quotation by Pearl Buck at the beginning of this chapter, there will never cease to be anxiety, agitation, unrest, and poor mental health until people are secure in the availability of adequate and healthy food. We all have a role in eliminating food insecurity as a socioenvironmental risk factor in the clinical setting and as a social determinant of poor mental health and mental illnesses in our communities and in society at large.

Key Points

- Food security is necessary for good mental health, and good mental health is important to one's ability to maintain food security. Food insecurity is clearly linked to depressive disorders and is likely linked to other specific mental illnesses, as well as one's general sense of well-being.

- Food insecurity is driven prominently by poverty or constrained financial resources. In the context of an abundant food supply in the United States, food insecurity commonly results in reduced dietary variety; low consumption of fresh fruits and vegetables and other micronutrient-rich foods; and increased intake of inexpensive, energy-dense, and nutritionally barren foods (thus leading to the association between food insecurity and overweight and obesity).

- Despite an abundant food supply, food insecurity is common in the United States, with roughly 15% of U.S. households being food insecure at some time during the year. Aside from outright food insecurity, even mild nutritional deficiencies have a negative impact on mental health.

- Mental health professionals receive little training on nutrition; however, they have an obligation to advise patients and their families about a healthy diet given that food-related risk factors can provoke and exacerbate mental illnesses. Mental health professionals who uncover food insecurity in a patient or family members can make appropriate referrals to local food banks and federal food and nutrition support programs.

- In addition to individual- and clinical-level interventions, policy approaches to food insecurity have a powerful effect on reducing food insecurity at the community and population levels. Important roles also exist for corporate America and citizens at large.

References

Alaimo K, Olson CM, Frongillo EA Jr: Food insufficiency and American school-aged children's cognitive, academic, and psychosocial development. Pediatrics 108(1):44–53, 2001 11433053

Alaimo K, Olson CM, Frongillo EA: Family food insufficiency, but not low family income, is positively associated with dysthymia and suicide symptoms in adolescents. J Nutr 132(4):719–725, 2002 11925467

Anderson SA: Core indicators of nutritional state for difficult-to-sample populations. J Nutr 120(Suppl 11):1559–1600, 1990 2243305

Bickel G, Nord M, Price C, et al: Guide to Measuring Household Food Security, Revised 2000. Alexandria, VA, U.S. Department of Agriculture, Food and Nutrition Service, March 2000

Bronte-Tinkew J, Zaslow M, Capps R, et al: Food insecurity works through depression, parenting, and infant feeding to influence overweight and health in toddlers. J Nutr 137(9):2160–2165, 2007 17709458

Burkhardt MC, Beck AF, Conway PH, et al: Enhancing accurate identification of food insecurity using quality-improvement techniques. Pediatrics 129(2):e504–e510, 2012

Chilton M, Rose D: A rights-based approach to food insecurity in the United States. Am J Public Health 99:1203–1211, 2009

Coleman-Jensen A, Nord M: Food Insecurity Among Households With Working-Age Adults With Disabilities (Economic Research Report No ERR-144). Washington, DC, U.S. Department of Agriculture, Economic Research Service, January 2013. Available at: http://www.ers.usda.gov/publications/err-economic-research-report/err144.aspx. Accessed April 24, 2013.

Coleman-Jensen A, Nord M, Andrews M, et al: Household Food Security in the United States in 2011 (Economic Research Report No ERR-141). Washington, DC, U.S. Department of Agriculture, Economic Research Service, September 2012. Available at: http://www.ers.usda.gov/media/884525/err141.pdf. Accessed April 24, 2013.

Compton MT, Daumit GL, Druss BG: Cigarette smoking and overweight/obesity among individuals with serious mental illnesses: a preventive perspective. Harv Rev Psychiatry 14(4):212–222, 2006 16912007

Cook JT, Frank DA, Berkowitz C, et al: Food insecurity is associated with adverse health outcomes among human infants and toddlers. J Nutr 134(6):1432–1438, 2004 15173408

Dinour LM, Bergen D, Yeh MC: The food insecurity-obesity paradox: a review of the literature and the role food stamps may play. J Am Diet Assoc 107(11):1952–1961, 2007 17964316

Feigelman S, Dubowitz H, Lane W, et al: Training pediatric residents in a primary care clinic to help address psychosocial problems and prevent child maltreatment. Acad Pediatr 11(6):474–480, 2011 21959095

Fleegler EW, Lieu TA, Wise PH, et al: Families' health-related social problems and missed referral opportunities. Pediatrics 119(6):e1332–e1341, 2007 17545363

Giang T, Karpyn A, Laurison HB, et al: Closing the grocery gap in underserved communities: the creation of the Pennsylvania Fresh Food Financing Initiative. J Public Health Manag Pract 14(3):272–279, 2008 18408552

Gittelsohn J, Song HJ, Suratkar S, et al: An urban food store intervention positively affects food-related psychosocial variables and food behaviors. Health Educ Behav 37(3):390–402, 2010 19887625

Gittelsohn J, Rowan M, Gadhoke P: Interventions in small food stores to change the food environment, improve diet, and reduce risk of chronic disease. Prev Chronic Dis 9:E59, 2012 22338599

Glanz K, Yaroch AL: Strategies for increasing fruit and vegetable intake in grocery stores and communities: policy, pricing, and environmental change. Prev Med 39(Suppl 2):S75–S80, 2004 15313075

Gowda C, Hadley C, Aiello AE: The association between food insecurity and inflammation in the US adult population. Am J Public Health 102(8):1579–1586, 2012 22698057

Gregory C, Ver Ploeg M, Andrews M, et al: Supplemental Nutrition Assistance Program (SNAP) Participation Leads to Modest Changes in Diet Quality (Economic Research Report No ERR-147). Washington, DC, U.S. Department of Agriculture, Economic Research Service, April 2013. http://www.ers.usda.gov/publications/err-economic-research-report/err147.aspx. Accessed February 4, 2014.

Hager ER, Quigg AM, Black MM, et al: Development and validity of a 2-item screen to identify families at risk for food insecurity. Pediatrics 126(1):e26–e32, 2010 20595453

Havens EK, Martin KS, Yan J, et al: Federal nutrition program changes and healthy food availability. Am J Prev Med 43(4):419–422, 2012 22992360

Heflin CM, Siefert K, Williams DR: Food insufficiency and women's mental health: findings from a 3-year panel of welfare recipients. Soc Sci Med 61(9):1971–1982, 2005 15927331

Hesecker H, Kübler W, Pudel V, et al: Psychological disorders as early symptoms of a mild-to-moderate vitamin deficiency. Ann N Y Acad Sci 669:352–357, 1992 1444045

Hoisington AT, Braverman MT, Hargunani DE, et al: Health care providers' attention to food insecurity in households with children. Prev Med 55(3):219–222, 2012 22710141

Hood C, Martinez-Donate A, Meinen A: Promoting healthy food consumption: a review of state-level policies to improve access to fruits and vegetables. WMJ 111(6):283–288, 2012 23362705

Hoyland A, Dye L, Lawton CL: A systematic review of the effect of breakfast on the cognitive performance of children and adolescents. Nutr Res Rev 22(2):220–243, 2009 19930787

Huddleston-Casas C, Charnigo R, Simmons LA: Food insecurity and maternal depression in rural, low-income families: a longitudinal investigation. Public Health Nutr 12(8):1133–1140, 2009 18789167

Institute of Medicine: Hunger and Obesity: Understanding a Food Insecurity Paradigm. Washington, DC, National Academies Press, 2011. Available at: http://iom.edu/Reports/2011/Hunger-and-Obesity-Understanding-a-Food-Insecurity-Paradigm.aspx. Accessed February 5, 2014.

Kirkpatrick SI, McIntyre L, Potestio ML: Child hunger and long-term adverse consequences for health. Arch Pediatr Adolesc Med 164(8):754–762, 2010 20679167

Kleinman RE, Murphy JM, Wieneke KM, et al: Use of a single-question screening tool to detect hunger in families attending a neighborhood health center. Ambul Pediatr 7(4):278–284, 2007 17660098

Laraia BA: Carrots, sticks, or carrot sticks?: using federal food policy to engineer dietary change. Am J Prev Med 43(4):456–457, 2012 22992366

Larson NI, Story MT: Food insecurity and weight status among U.S. children and families: a review of the literature. Am J Prev Med 40(2):166–173, 2011 21238865

Larson NI, Story MT, Nelson MC: Neighborhood environments: disparities in access to healthy foods in the U.S. Am J Prev Med 36(1):74–81, 2009 18977112

Lent MD, Petrovic LE, Swanson JA, et al: Maternal mental health and the persistence of food insecurity in poor rural families. J Health Care Poor Underserved 20(3):645–661, 2009 19648695

Ludwig DS, Blumenthal SJ, Willett WC: Opportunities to reduce childhood hunger and obesity: restructuring the Supplemental Nutrition Assistance Program (the Food Stamp Program). JAMA 308(24):2567–2568, 2012 23268513

McElroy SL, Kotwal R, Malhotra S, et al: Are mood disorders and obesity related? A review for the mental health professional. J Clin Psychiatry 65(5):634–651, quiz 730, 2004 15163249

McLaughlin I, Kramer K: Food retailer licensing: an innovative approach to increasing access to healthful foods. Prev Chronic Dis 9:E170, 2012 23194778

Nestle M: Food Politics: How the Food Industry Influences Nutrition and Health. Berkeley, University of California Press, 2002

Oliveira V: The Food Assistance Landscape: FY 2011 Annual Report (EIB-93). Washington, DC, U.S. Department of Agriculture, Economic Research Service, 2012. Available at: http://www.ers.usda.gov/media/376910/eib93_1_.pdf. Accessed April 24, 2013.

Robertson A, Brunner E, Sheiham A: Food is a political issue, in Social Determinants of Mental Health, 2nd Edition. Edited by Marmot M, Wilkinson RG. Oxford, UK, Oxford University Press, 2006, pp 172–195

Sabia JJ: The effect of body weight on adolescent academic performance. South Econ J 73(4):871–900, 2007

Seligman HK, Laraia BA, Kushel MB: Food insecurity is associated with chronic disease among low-income NHANES participants. J Nutr 140(2):304–310, 2010 20032485

Seligman HK, Jacobs EA, López A, et al: Food insecurity and glycemic control among low-income patients with type 2 diabetes. Diabetes Care 35(2):233–238, 2012 22210570

Siefert K, Heflin CM, Corcoran ME, et al: Food insufficiency and the physical and mental health of low-income women. Women Health 32(1–2):159–177, 2001 11459368

Stang J, Taft Bayerl C, Flatt MM, et al: Position of the American Dietetic Association: child and adolescent food and nutrition programs. J Am Diet Assoc 106(9):1467–1475, 2006 16986233

Stuff JE, Casey PH, Szeto KL, et al: Household food insecurity is associated with adult health status. J Nutr 134(9):2330–2335, 2004 15333724

U.S. Department of Agriculture, U.S. Department of Health and Human Services: Dietary Guidelines for Americans, 2010, 7th Edition. Washington, DC, U.S. Government Printing Office, December 2010

Walker RE, Keane CR, Burke JG: Disparities and access to healthy food in the United States: a review of food deserts literature. Health Place 16(5):876–884, 2010 20462784

Whitaker RC, Phillips SM, Orzol SM: Food insecurity and the risks of depression and anxiety in mothers and behavior problems in their preschool-aged children. Pediatrics 118(3):e859–e868, 2006 16950971

Wilkinson R, Pickett K: The Spirit Level: Why Greater Equality Makes Societies Stronger. New York: Bloomsbury Press, 2009

Wolfe WS, Olson CM, Kendall A, et al: Hunger and food insecurity in the elderly: its nature and measurement. J Aging Health 10(3):327–350, 1998 10342935

World Health Organization: Food Security (World Health Organization Web site), 2014. Available at: http://www.who.int/trade/glossary/story028/en/. Accessed April 16, 2014.

Wunderlich G, Norwood J (eds): National Research Council: Food Insecurity in the United States: An Assessment of the Measure. Panel to Review the US Department of Agriculture's Measurement of Food Insecurity and Hunger. Washington, DC, National Academies Press, 2006

Zaslow M, Bronte-Tinkew J, Capps R, et al: Food security during infancy: implications for attachment and mental proficiency in toddlerhood. Matern Child Health J 13(1):66–80, 2009 18317892

Zenk SN, Odoms-Young A, Powell LM, et al: Fruit and vegetable availability and selection: federal food package revisions, 2009. Am J Prev Med 43(4):423–428, 2012 22992361

8

Poor Housing Quality and Housing Instability

Shakira F. Suglia, Sc.D., M.S.
Earle Chambers, Ph.D., M.P.H.
Megan T. Sandel, M.D., M.P.H.

The connection between health and the dwelling of the population is one of the most important that exists.

Florence Nightingale, 1820–1910

Housing is a fundamental necessity. In the most basic sense, housing provides shelter from the elements and supports the storage of food and water. Housing is much more than shelter, however, because it provides a place for family and community gathering, it evokes a sense of stability and security, and it provides a sense of identity. As a correlate of an individual's socioeconomic status, great variation in the type, size, and quality of housing exists, which can have major implications for health. Housing affects health through structural, psychological, and social pathways (Dunn 2002; Shaw 2004). As noted by Shaw (2004), inadequate housing conditions are associated with both physical and mental illnesses through direct and indirect pathways (Figure 8–1). Structural features of the home (e.g., mold, pest infestation, peeling paint, crowding) directly impact health, whereas location (e.g., accessibility to services and facilities), neighborhood built environment (e.g., availability of recreational facilities and parks, walkability), and social connectedness to a community indirectly affect health (Shaw 2004).

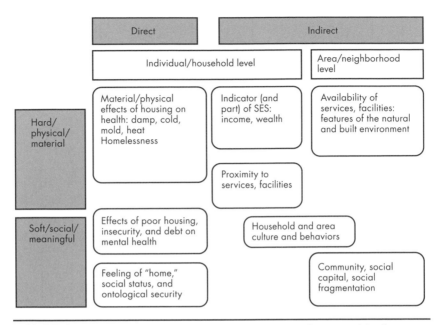

FIGURE 8-1.   Conceptual model depicting the direct and indirect relation between housing and health.

SES=socioeconomic status.

Source.   Reprinted from Shaw M: "Housing and Public Health." *Annual Review of Public Health* 25:397–418, 2004. Used with permission.

In this chapter, we conceptualize housing conditions and the presence or absence of stable housing as a public health problem and a determinant of mental health. Although housing and neighborhood are closely linked together, we focus on the relation between housing per se and mental health problems; the topic of adverse features of the built environment as a social determinant of mental health is discussed in Chapter 9, "Adverse Features of the Built Environment."

Defining Poor Housing Quality and Housing Instability

Several housing-related constructs have been defined in the literature and examined for their relation to mental health, such as housing deterioration or quality, structural characteristics of the home, housing instability or insecurity, home ownership, affordability, and homelessness.

Much of the existing research focuses on housing instability and poor housing quality as determinants of mental health; other constructs less widely examined are perceptions of the housing environment and structural characteristics of the home not related to quality.

The literature has some variation as to the definition of housing instability. Commonly, housing instability is defined as two or more moves in 1 year. Other definitions of housing instability are more closely tied with episodes of homelessness, such as spending a night at a shelter or in a car within a defined period of time. Standard measures have been developed to assess housing structural conditions, enabling the characterization of housing quality as adequate or inadequate (Table 8–1). For example, the American Housing Survey has developed a series of questions to assess physical housing conditions (U.S. Census Bureau 2014). Other epidemiological studies (e.g., the Fragile Families and Child Wellbeing Study) have adapted these questions to more comprehensively assess the integrity of the physical home environment (e.g., whether the home unit contains broken windows or cracked windowpanes, open cracks or holes in walls or ceiling, holes in the floor, broken or falling plaster, peeling paint, frayed electrical wires, mice or rats, broken glass, broken stairs, and other hazards). Other housing characteristics that are not structural are less often assessed, yet they have been shown to also affect mental health. For example, the Fragile Families and Child Wellbeing Study, a population-based study of a sample of disadvantaged urban women, assessed, in addition to the physical integrity of the home, variables pertaining to the organization of the home environment (e.g., if the inside of the home is dark or crowded, if it is cluttered or dirty or not reasonably clean, if the house is overly noisy because of inside or outside noise). Housing quality items discussed in the Fragile Families and Child Wellbeing Study are consistent with items from previous work on housing conditions demonstrating links to psychological distress (Evans et al. 2000b; Sandel and Wright 2006; Shaw 2004).

Perceptions of or satisfaction with the housing environment have also been explored (e.g., fear of eviction, inability to contact one's landlord, lack of control over repairs, affordability). The perceptions and satisfaction construct, although less often assessed, has been associated with a sense of lack of control over one's own housing situation and thus is more directly linked to perceptions of stress and negative emotional responses. Structural features of the home, such as the age of the home, whether it is a high-rise or low-rise dwelling, and whether it is a single-unit or multiunit home, have also been assessed to determine their relation to physical and mental health outcomes. Future assessments of

TABLE 8–1.	Sample items commonly used to define housing quality, instability, perceptions, and structural features of the home

Housing deterioration
    Open cracks in walls
    Holes in floors
    Home hard to heat
    Cold house for 24 hours or more last winter
    Presence of rats, mice, or cockroaches
    Presence of water leaks or mold
    Peeling paint or plaster
Housing instability
    Number of moves in the past year
    Sleeping in a car or shelter
    Having to stay at friends' or family's house
Housing perceptions
    Crowded living conditions
    Desire to move from the area
    Fear of eviction
    Loud street noise or noise from heavy traffic
    Difficulty contacting landlord
    Hard to get landlord to fix things
Housing structural characteristics
    Multi-unit versus single-unit housing
    Age of the home
    Number of people living in the home and number of rooms

housing conditions should include a broad range of questions that capture the many dimensions of housing. In addition to independently rated measures of housing quality, subjective perceptions of housing quality should also be assessed to provide a more comprehensive picture of housing quality as it relates to mental health.

These constructs (housing quality, instability, structural characteristics, and perceptions) are not completely independent factors; however, they have been examined in the literature separately and might have differential effects on physical and mental health. They are also associated with other social determinants of physical and mental health. For example, housing instability has been associated with other social determinants, such as food insecurity (Cutts et al. 2011). Given the existing evidence, it can be hypothesized that the effects of experiencing multiple housing stressors, such as both housing instability and poor housing quality, are more detrimental to health than the effect of experiencing only one.

Poor Housing Quality and Housing Instability as Social Determinants of Health

It is estimated that 35 million homes in the United States are characterized by inadequate living conditions (e.g., they are structurally deteriorated, crowded, or hazardous), and more than 600,000 people are homeless on any given night in the United States (National Alliance to End Homelessness 2013; National Center for Healthy Housing 2013). Housing conditions are tied to economic factors at both the individual level and the neighborhood level; thus, housing quality differs greatly by individual socioeconomic status, with lower socioeconomic status and racial and ethnic minorities being more likely to experience housing instability and poor housing quality than other groups. Geographic location is the second largest determinant of housing conditions. Age of the housing stock, for example, is greatly determined by geographic location, and older housing may require more maintenance, expose residents to environmental pollutants (e.g., lead), and be less energy efficient. State and local policies, which define and enforce the standards by which housing should be kept, also vary by region.

Poor housing quality and housing instability have been associated with numerous physical health conditions, including respiratory conditions due primarily to poor indoor air quality, cognitive delays in children from exposure to neurotoxins (e.g., lead), and accidents and injuries as a result of structural deficiencies. The social and mental health consequences of poor housing quality and instability have also been noted. Housing instability disrupts work, school, and day care arrangements, as well as social networks of both parents and children. Worries over the stability of one's housing situation and poor control over the conditions of one's home can result in distress and subsequent mental disorders. Children and adults experience poor housing quality and instability differently, with further variations among children depending on their developmental stage.

Poor Housing Quality and Housing Instability as Social Determinants of Mental Health

Impact of Poor Housing Quality and Housing Instability on Adults

As shown in Table 8–2, four different types of housing factors have been examined in relation to mental health among adults: 1) structural features of the home, such as type of dwelling (high rise vs. low rise) and floor level (high vs. low); 2) housing quality (e.g., pest infestation, mold, dampness, deterioration); 3) housing instability, defined as frequent moves or, in its most extreme form, homelessness; and 4) housing perceptions (e.g., control over repairs, housing costs, overcrowding).

Specific structural features of the home have been associated with psychological health (Weich et al. 2002). For example, living in a multiunit dwelling, on a higher floor level, and in a high-rise apartment building have been associated with distress symptoms and depression among women (Evans et al. 2003). Structural features of the home are hypothesized to affect mental health by restricting social interactions with neighbors and causing social isolation. Compared with working adults, elderly persons who spend more time at home and have fewer opportunities for social interactions outside of the home may be more vulnerable to such structural features of the home environment that restrict social connections.

A relation between poor housing quality and mental health is thought to be partly attributable to the fact that issues affecting housing quality are perceived as stressors that are proximal or immediate and largely out of one's control (Miller and Rasmussen 2010). Features of housing quality, such as structural deterioration of the home, presence of mold, and pest infestation, are associated with distress (Sandel and Wright 2006; Shenassa et al. 2007). Shenassa and colleagues (2007) examined the relation between dampness or mold in the home and depression using survey data from eight European cities. Dampness or mold in the home was associated with depression; however, the associations became attenuated after adjustment for perception of control, indicating that perceived control might mediate the relation. The link between structural deterioration of the home and mental well-being could be due to various factors, such as difficulties in dealing with needed repairs and landlords, the stigma attached to living in a deteri-

TABLE 8–2.   Some of the associations documented between housing constructs and adult and child mental health outcomes

Housing construct	Adult mental health outcomes	Child mental health outcomes
Structural factors	Depression	Anxiety Behavioral problems (hyperactivity, hostility) Juvenile delinquency
Poor quality	Psychological distress Depression Poor general mental health Anxiety	Problems with social adaptation
Instability	Depression Anxiety	Emotional and school problems Internalizing and externalizing behaviors
Perceptions (disarray, problems paying bills)	Poor mental health Depression Anxiety	

orated home, and concerns about being evicted (Evans 2003; Evans et al. 2003). Less is known about other factors (e.g., water leaks) as they relate to mental health.

Episodes of homelessness have also been associated, unsurprisingly, with poor mental and physical health (Grant et al. 2013; Munoz et al. 2005). Physical and mental health problems are often also an antecedent to homelessness because they can interfere with one's ability to work and can deplete economic resources (Wells et al. 2010). In addition, mental health problems can isolate individuals, leaving them with less social support and putting them at greater risk for homelessness. For the majority of the U.S. population that experiences homelessness, the experience is brief; however, 17% of the total homeless population is chronically homeless (Bauer et al. 2013). Chronic homelessness, defined as being homeless continuously for 1 year or having at least four episodes of homelessness in a 3-year period, is clearly associated with mental illnesses (Fazel et al. 2008). Although homelessness can cause distress and exacerbate an existing mental illness, having a mental illness is also a major risk factor for homelessness. Difficulties in maintaining a job, low wages, and lack of resources make it more likely for those with mental disorders to experience homelessness; being homeless, in turn, can exacerbate mental disorders, including substance use disorders. Not only are homeless persons exposed to more stressors and adverse living conditions, but for those who have a mental disorder, not having a secure place to live makes it more difficult to seek care, follow up with services, and afford and adhere to medications (Bauer et al. 2013). Thus, the relation between chronic homelessness and poor mental health is cyclical, making it particularly difficult to address.

Frequent moves, a lower-intensity stressor, may also generate psychological distress. In longitudinal studies, residential instability—defined as frequently moving or not having enough money to pay rent—has been associated with depression among women (Davey-Rothwell et al. 2008; Magdol 2002). In a study of people who abuse substances and their social network members, Davey-Rothwell and colleagues (2008) noted that frequent moves in a 6-month period were associated with higher levels of depressive symptoms, independent of homelessness in the past 6 months. Thus, although mental health problems can lead to housing instability, housing instability can also be a precursor for mental health problems; the linkages are bidirectional. In one study, the influence of housing quality and instability on mental health (depression and generalized anxiety disorder) was examined among women participating in the Fragile Families and Child Wellbeing Study (Suglia et al. 2011). Analyses accounted for two social factors: intimate partner violence and financial hardship. In the sample of approximately 2,000 women, 16% were classified as having probable depression, and 5% were classified as having probable generalized anxiety disorder. In adjusted analyses, mothers experiencing housing disarray (e.g., dark, crowded, noisy housing) and instability (i.e., moving more than twice in the past year) were more likely to screen positive for depression (odds ratio [OR] 1.3, 95% confidence interval [CI] 1.0–1.7 and OR 1.4, 95% CI 1.2–2.3, respectively). In addition, those experiencing housing instability were more likely to screen positive for generalized anxiety disorder (OR 1.9, 95% CI 1.2–3.0) even after adjusting for other social factors. Other studies have found housing instability to be associated with poor mental health (Davey-Rothwell et al. 2008; Magdol 2002; Matheson et al. 2006). Housing instability could affect mental health through several pathways. Constant moves disturb social networks and can result in more isolation, lack of access to support and family, and less access to health care. Housing instability can also disrupt children's routines, day care, and school arrangements, which could lead to more distress among mothers (Suglia et al. 2011).

Housing features not related to structure, quality, or instability have also been linked to psychological distress. For example, housing costs and perceived lack of control over housing (e.g., having a landlord who is unavailable to carry out repairs) have been associated with distress symptoms and poor mental health (Dunn 2002; Dunn and Hayes 1999; Evans et al. 2000a). Further evidence supporting the relation between housing and mental health is the fact that improvement of housing conditions and moving to better-quality housing have been demonstrated to improve mental health outcomes (Elton and Packer 1986; Halpern 1995).

Impact of Poor Housing Quality and Housing Instability on Children

Worries about the quality or stability of housing can adversely affect not only adult mental health but also parent-child interactions and, ultimately, child mental health. Structural features of the home can make it difficult for parents to supervise children and can restrict children's and adolescents' opportunities to interact with peers. Frequent moves can result in changing care and school routines and disturb social networks for both children and their parents. Few studies have examined features of the housing environment and mental health outcomes among children, but they have found that frequent moves, adverse structural features of the home, and housing instability affect school achievement, social and emotional adjustment, child behavior, and adolescent mental health (Leventhal and Newman 2010).

Stability in a child's life provides the structure and consistency necessary for emotional development. Housing instability disrupts school and care routines, fragments social networks, and upsets a sense of security and consistency necessary for optimal child development. Several studies have examined the role of housing instability in shaping emotional and behavioral disorders in children (Adam and Chase-Lansdale 2002; Wood et al. 1993). Recently, using data from the Fragile Families and Child Wellbeing Study, Ziol-Guest and McKenna (2014) noted that moving three or more times in a child's first 5 years of life is significantly associated with attention problems, as well as internalizing and externalizing behavioral problems, but only among poor children. Families of lower socioeconomic status have fewer resources and thus may be more vulnerable to housing disruptions. Additionally, in a longitudinal study using data from the National Survey of Child and Adolescent Well-Being, the effects of housing mobility were noted to depend on the age of the child at the time of the exposure. Children 4–6 years of age who experienced frequent moves in the previous 12 months exhibited higher levels of externalizing behaviors that persisted over time, yet no effects were noted among school-age children. Among adolescents 11–14 years of age, frequent moves were associated with increased behavioral problems across a 3-year follow-up (Fowler et al. 2014). These data lend insights into the mechanisms associated with housing instability and behavior. As the authors hypothesized, preschool-age children, who may be spending more time at home relative to time spent at home by school-age children, may be exposed to higher levels of family dysfunction. The noted association between frequent moves and behavioral problems in adolescents may be a consequence of the disruption of their social networks compared with younger school-age children.

Only a few studies have examined the quality of the home environment as a determinant of child mental health. Structural features such as high-rise dwellings have been associated with more behavioral problems among children, a connection thought to be due to restricted play opportunities and limited social interactions with other children (Evans 2003).

In summary, studies have shown that specific features of one's housing are related to mental health even after adjusting for social stressors. Particularly for young mothers and their children, providing resources to obtain and maintain adequate housing would be beneficial to both mother and child because housing conditions have been shown to affect both physical and mental health (Evans 2006). In addition to being directly affected by housing conditions, children could be indirectly affected by their caretakers' mental health status, which is also affected by housing conditions. Thus, addressing and eliminating stressors experienced by caretakers, such as poor housing quality, can potentially benefit the parent's as well as the child's health and well-being.

Poor Housing Quality and Housing Instability in the Clinical Setting

As previously noted, both inadequate and unaffordable housing can affect the mental health and well-being of both adults and children. Health care professionals can advocate for healthy and secure housing for their patients by partnering with legal, public health, and housing services. Creating access to housing inspections and legal services in the health care setting can be an effective way of addressing mental health risks related to the home.

Case Example: A Lack of Healthy and Safe Housing in the Context of Emotional Stress

Dr. Roberta Carlson is a pediatric pulmonologist at a public health clinic in an impoverished area of a large city. She and her colleagues primarily treat low-income children receiving public insurance. Jaclyn Richards, age 30, brings her 12-year-old daughter, Kyla Richards, to receive ongoing treatment of previously diagnosed asthma from Dr. Carlson.

Kyla has been in treatment for asthma for 6 years. Her asthma seems to be triggered by dust, cold air, exercise, and emotional stress. Ms. Richards first brought Kyla to Dr. Carlson when she was 6 years old. Dr. Carlson explained that Kyla's asthma is triggered by dust and that it is best for her to live in a dust-free environment. She advised Ms. Richards on ways to avoid exposing Kyla to dust, including the use of dust covers on the bed. The family also received visits from a community health worker, who reinforced the importance of medication adherence and helped Ms. Richards identify and remediate triggers and select appropriate cleaning materials.

Kyla's health improved after these interventions, and she experienced a long period of symptom stability. However, a few months ago, she developed increased asthma attacks. Dr. Carlson treated her with a short taper of oral prednisone, and she seemed to respond well. Now, Kyla has quickly developed recurrent wheezing. She also has been sleeping poorly because of increasing respiratory symptoms and needs another short course of prednisone.

Although it seems feasible for Dr. Carlson to advise the family about reducing exposure to allergens, a more difficult task is addressing the emotional stress created by Kyla's home and neighborhood conditions. Dr. Carlson can inquire about Kyla's living situation and investigate if features of the family's housing might be affecting Kyla's health. The following questions are of particular interest: Has anything happened within Kyla's home that might be causing emotional stress, which could then trigger her asthma? Do Ms. Richards and Kyla feel safe at home? Is violence a concern for them? Do they ever struggle to pay rent or utility bills? Who lives with them?

After asking about their housing situation, Dr. Carlson learns that Kyla and Ms. Richards live in a local public housing development. Their apartment has a leaking pipe, and Ms. Richards is having difficulty getting someone to fix it. The leak is causing mold, which could be worsening Kyla's asthma. Ms. Richards feels stressed about the mold, and Kyla has witnessed her crying in her bedroom. Recently, Ms. Richards's sister lost her job, and she and her two children have been living in Ms. Richards's one-bedroom apartment. The day after hearing gunshots in the street outside her home, Kyla learned that one of her peers had been fatally shot. She has been experiencing severe asthma symptoms ever since hearing this news.

After learning more about Kyla's home environment, Dr. Carlson can now work with legal, public health, and mental health professionals to address issues such as overcrowded housing and violence that are affecting Kyla's emotional health and, in turn, worsening her physical health. The emotional stress caused by her home situation, along with the physical housing issues of mold and overcrowding, may have contributed to Kyla experiencing an exacerbation of asthma. In addition, in a circular effect, the experience of having an asthma attack also causes her to feel anxious and frightened that it might happen again.

Assessing Poor Housing Quality and Housing Instability in the Clinical Setting

Health care providers can be trained by attorneys and paralegal professionals, specifically through a medical-legal partnership, to screen for social determinants of health, including housing-related social determinants. As shown in Table 8–3, health care professionals can also use the assessment tool I-HELP (income, housing, education, legal status, literacy, and personal safety) (Kenyon et al. 2007) to identify patients' concerns that might have a legal remedy, including housing problems. For example, to determine if there is a violation of sanitary code, a physician might ask, "Do you ever see cockroaches or mice?" Research shows that the type of housing (owner-occupied, rental, or public housing) can have effects on mental health. Thus, health care providers can ask, for example, "Do you rent or own your home?" Electronic medical records can prompt health care providers to ask about housing issues and concerns.

However, it is a much simpler task to identify the problems and connections between negative health outcomes and inadequate housing than it is to fix them. Given the difficulty and hesitance of renters to navigate the legal system, it is beneficial for health care communities to collaborate with legal, housing, and public health services to advocate for safe and health-promoting housing and legal assistance when necessary.

How Clinicians Can Address Poor Housing Quality and Housing Instability

Many housing concerns are legal in nature, and the law can be useful and is often necessary to secure safe and stable housing for individuals and families. Programs that provide housing to the most vulnerable homeless populations have been demonstrated to be effective in improving

TABLE 8–3. Examples of potential social history questions using the I-HELP mnemonic

Domain or area	Examples of questions
Income	
General	Do you ever have trouble making ends meet?
Food income	Do you ever have a time when you don't have enough food? Do you have WIC? Food stamps?
Housing	
Housing	Is your housing ever a problem for you?
Utilities	Do you ever have trouble paying your electric/heat/telephone bill?
Education	
Appropriate education placement	How is your child doing in school? Is he or she getting the help to learn what he or she needs?
Early childhood program	Is your child in Head Start, preschool, or other early childhood enrichment?
Legal status	
Immigration	Do you have questions about your immigration status? Do you need help accessing benefits or services for your family?
Literacy	
Child literacy	Do you read to your child every night?
Parent literacy	How happy are you with how you read?
Personal safety	
Domestic violence	Have you ever taken out a restraining order? Do you feel safe in your relationship?
General safety	Do you feel safe in your home? In your neighborhood?

Note. WIC=Special Supplemental Nutrition Program for Women, Infants, and Children.

Source. Reprinted from Kenyon C, Sandel M, Silverstein M, et al.: "Revisiting the Social History for Child Health." *Pediatrics* 120(3):e734–e738, 2007. Used with permission.

mental health and housing outcomes. Examples of such programs include the housing-first model, which seeks to move homeless individuals or households immediately from the streets or homeless shelters into their own apartments, with an ultimate longer-term goal of independent housing (Rynearson et al. 2010), and supportive housing, which provides a range of approaches that aim to provide safe, stable, and supported housing for persons with psychiatric disabilities (Cheng et al. 2007). State and local housing codes regulate the construction and condition of residential properties and ensure safe and healthy housing. It is illegal for landlords to ignore these codes. For example, sanitary codes require that residential owners maintain proper kitchen facilities, hot water, and adequate heat and lighting. The exact nature of these codes varies between states and municipalities, and enforcement is the responsibility of public agencies that perform inspections in addition to housing courts. Unsafe housing conditions such as mold and pest infestation that can result in poorer mental health can also represent an unlawful violation of tenant rights. Therefore, enforcement of environmental and housing-related laws can serve as both a preventive and therapeutic approach for patients and also improve social justice by reducing disparities.

Tenants have the right to complain to state and local code enforcement agencies when landlords do not address violations. However, low-income tenants living in substandard housing are not always aware of their right to a safe and healthy home. Defending one's right to adequate housing often requires ample financial resources, legal information, time, and energy, which are often scarce among poor and disadvantaged people. Therefore, health care providers can work to increase access to legal services in order to ensure safe and secure housing for their patients.

Utilizing legal and housing organizations to improve housing might also lead to an enhanced sense of control among patients. The frequent communication and trust within the health care community, combined with the impact of housing problems on mental health, make medical settings an ideal place to enable access to legal aid. The following three models have been successful in establishing effective communication and advocacy between families, health care teams, and legal professionals to improve housing for patients.

The *medical-legal partnership* (MLP) model brings legal aid into the health care setting or to medical homes. MLP joins clinical and legal staff to identify and correct barriers to health, including housing violations. In some housing cases, legal advice or representation might be needed to advocate for residents. Landlords sometimes avoid their responsibilities of following codes that require safe and healthy housing until they are threatened with legal action. If needed, patients are referred to an on-site MLP lawyer who works to enforce the patient's rights and to help meet the individual's or family's basic needs.

Clinicians, including mental health professionals, can use legal form letters, designed specifically for providers, to ask landlords to change unfit housing conditions. Lawyers can both advise their clients to act within the guidelines of the law and, when necessary, place demands on landlord and management companies to deal with unfavorable housing conditions. MLP staff can also help patients get higher priorities on waitlists for benefits such as housing subsidies.

The *Breathe Easy at Home* (BEAH) program in Boston is an example of an effective collaboration between legal, public health, and clinical services. The BEAH program brings together several agencies within the city of Boston, including the Inspectional Services Department's Housing Inspection Division, Boston Medical Center, Boston Public Health Commission, and local community health centers. This program allows health care professionals to refer patients for housing inspections if they suspect substandard housing conditions. It was developed to ensure that inspections, where warranted, are performed quickly and that any follow-up inspections are conducted to ensure that substandard conditions are resolved. By utilizing a shared Web site, health care professionals can track children through the inspection, violation reparation, reinspection, and housing court processes. Using a shared Web site also improves communication between the medical, public health, and housing communities in hopes of reducing substandard conditions so that children can be healthier (Reid et al. 2014). In a pilot evaluation study, families who participated in BEAH reported a general overall improvement in health.

Another approach is the *community health worker* model. Housing residents themselves play a key role in maintaining safe and healthy living spaces. In some cases, individuals' smoking habits or housekeeping practices might be making the home detrimental to mental health. Health care teams can incorporate home visitors or community health workers to deliver tenant education within the home. Such community health workers can walk through the home and determine specific steps that residents can take to improve their housing conditions. They can also provide education, healthy home supplies such as trash cans and sealed food containers, and smoking cessation referrals.

Linking clinical settings with public health, housing, and legal assistance provides a way for clinicians to better ensure that their patients' housing needs are met. Because low-income renters are often not accustomed to accessing the legal system to secure safe and healthy housing but are accustomed to frequently utilizing the health care system, health care providers can play a key role in ensuring healthy and secure housing. These collaborations can be very effective in documenting and addressing the health effects of substandard housing.

Policy Approaches to Poor Housing Quality and Housing Instability

Although existing evidence points to a consistent association between several housing parameters and mental health, few studies have examined housing policies and related physical or mental health outcomes. Housing policies in the United States have been enacted not to address physical and mental health needs but to attend to a shortage of affordable housing. Unfortunately, some of these housing programs have had unintended consequences. The development of public housing in resource-poor neighborhoods, for example, has worsened racial and economic residential segregation, locating greater numbers of racial/ethnic minorities and the poor in neighborhoods that have fewer resources for optimal well-being. This segregation places people in areas of concentrated poverty, which is detrimental to physical and mental well-being.

Local and State Policy and Programs Affecting Housing

The Chicago Housing Authority's Plan for Transformation serves as one example of a local housing program aimed at improving housing conditions at a community level while at the same time improving the overall health of residents (Popkin et al. 2013). After decades of management neglect, physically hazardous conditions, crime, and vandalism in Chicago's high-rise public housing towers, in 1999, the Chicago Housing Authority launched a Plan for Transformation to convert its properties into healthy, mixed-income communities (Cunningham et al. 2005). Central to the plan for transformation was the relocation of residents, which involved intensive case management and referral services. After several years, a substantial number of "hard-to-house residents" who did not meet the criteria for new mixed-income housing or vouchers were unable to relocate and thus remained living in conditions that were increasingly deteriorating as the developments emptied out (Cunningham et al. 2005). In 2005, the Housing Authority partnered with the Urban Institute, Heartland Human Care Services, and Housing Choice Partners to provide intensive services for the left-behind families (Cunningham et al. 2005). This rigorous Chicago Family Case Management Demonstration project involved mental health counseling, substance abuse treatment, transitional jobs, financial literacy workshops, and enhanced mobility counseling. Evaluation of the demonstration project revealed significant gains in employment for working-age participants and improved mental and physical health. Demonstration project participants were significantly less likely to report symptoms of depression in 2011 compared with 2007 and were less likely to report anxiety between 2009 and 2011 (Popkin et al. 2013). Unfortunately, the youth who lived through the Housing Authority's Plan for Transformation did not benefit; an evaluation of the project demonstrated that teens were still struggling with academic failure, delinquency, and trauma (Popkin et al. 2013). A lack of directed services to youth highlights the need for intensive and targeted interventions.

Federal Policy and Programs Affecting Housing

One federal program that exists to address the affordability of housing is the Low Income Housing Tax Credits program, an indirect subsidy that helps to finance the development of affordable rental housing for low-income households. Public housing facilities, intended to address affordability, are often of poorer quality; that is, they are often substandard in ways that affect residents' health. Furthermore, they often are located in neighborhoods characterized by concentrated poverty. Although aiming to address housing affordability, they expose families to detrimental neighborhood factors, thus erasing many potential health gains of affordable housing. To partly address these issues, the federal Section 8 Housing Choice Voucher program allows low-income families to move into mixed-income housing without an increase in their rental burden beyond what they would pay in public housing. A few studies have attempted to evaluate the health and well-being benefits of this voucher-based housing program among low-income residents who are able to relocate to a mixed-income option. The underlying theory is that mixed-income neighborhoods provide to low-income families a number of social resources (e.g., social norms and networks that promote a healthier lifestyle) and material resources (e.g., better access to healthy food options and places to be physically active) that are not available in areas of concentrated poverty. When low-income families move to these mixed-income neighborhoods, it is thought that they are better able to prioritize healthy behaviors not only because the neighborhood supports these behaviors but because they have a rental burden that is not consistent with the market rate in that area and thus have more disposable income to afford healthy options.

The Moving to Opportunity (MTO) study, initiated by the U.S. Department of Housing and Urban Development, was a randomized study in five large U.S. cities (Baltimore, Boston, Chicago, Los Angeles, and New York) that examined the benefits of using Section 8 vouchers to move families out of housing projects and into mixed-income housing (Kling et al. 2007; U.S. Department of Housing and Urban Development 1996). In the experimental group, families were voluntarily relocated into mixed-income housing that accepted Section 8 vouchers in low-poverty neighborhoods. The control group included those who stayed in public housing. A recent follow-up of MTO participants noted better mental health outcomes among mothers in the treatment group. Among youth, however, the results were mixed. Beneficial mental health effects were noted among adolescent girls but not adolescent boys (Kessler et al. 2014). The MTO study was unable to characterize the built and social environment that participants lived in, making it difficult to identify mechanisms that could explain why Section 8 housing conferred better mental health outcomes to mothers and young girls specifically.

Despite the limited evidence elucidating which housing policies best influence health outcomes, general support exists for the idea that affordable housing options have many benefits that ultimately influence health. The current evidence suggests differential health benefits for different populations and suggests more supportive services may be needed for specific subgroups. Thus, in addition to partnerships that address poor housing quality and housing instability in the clinical setting, clinicians, including mental health professionals, can have a role in policy discussions pertaining to affordable and safe housing. Such efforts are likely to promote health and reduce the risk of both physical and mental illnesses.

Promoting Safe and Secure Housing: A Role for Everyone

Housing and mental health are connected. On the one hand, adverse housing conditions can prompt or exacerbate existing mental health problems among residents. On the other, the presence of poor mental health or mental illnesses can make maintaining stable housing difficult. Fortunately, evidence shows that housing-related policies coupled with clinical strategies to manage mental health, which include advocating for better housing conditions for at-risk patients, can reduce the risk of adverse mental health outcomes. Local and federal policies are necessary to address the housing issues and difficulties related to access to resources that accompany concentrated-poverty environments, including those with racial and economic residential segregation. The MTO and similar studies, as well as the work of MLP and other partnerships, suggest that housing policies that increase access to healthful resources can be coupled with targeted individual-level efforts to increase mental well-being among residents.

Although policy makers clearly have a major role in improving the quality of housing and minimizing housing instability, mental health professionals and other clinicians can also actively participate. More broadly, every citizen can be involved by becoming more knowledgeable of the health effects of housing; making voting decisions that are informed about housing policy; and participating in the discourse on ensuring high-quality, safe, secure, and healthy housing for all citizens.

Key Points

- Poor housing quality and housing instability are major public health concerns, affecting both physical and mental health outcomes among adults and children.

- Elderly populations, as well as young mothers and children who spend more time in the home, may be particularly vulnerable to the adverse effects of poor housing quality.

- Clinicians can identify housing problems and other social problems that affect physical and mental health with a very brief assessment and can work with existing programs such as a medical-legal partnership to aid patients in solving housing problems by accessing available legal resources when necessary.

- An examination of current housing policies at the state and federal level is needed to determine the effect of existing policies on physical and mental health. Any interventions to relocate residents should be accompanied by targeted interventions to address the many physical and mental health issues that affect vulnerable populations.

References

Adam EK, Chase-Lansdale PL: Home sweet home(s): parental separations, residential moves, and adjustment problems in low-income adolescent girls. Dev Psychol 38(5):792–805, 2002 12220056

Bauer LK, Baggett TP, Stern TA, et al: Caring for homeless persons with serious mental illness in general hospitals. Psychosomatics 54(1):14–21, 2013 23295004

Cheng AL, Lin H, Kasprow W, et al: Impact of supported housing on clinical outcomes: analysis of a randomized trial using multiple imputation technique. J Nerv Ment Dis 195(1):83–88, 2007 17220745

Cunningham MK, Popkin SJ, Burt MR: Public Housing Transformation and the "Hard to House." Washington, DC, Urban Institute, 2005. Available at: http://www.urban.org/UploadedPDF/311178_Roof_9.pdf. Accessed April 27, 2014.

Cutts DB, Meyers AF, Black MM, et al: US housing insecurity and the health of very young children. Am J Public Health 101(8):1508–1514, 2011 21680929

Davey-Rothwell MA, German D, Latkin CA: Residential transience and depression: does the relationship exist for men and women? J Urban Health 85(5):707–716, 2008 18581237

Dunn JR: Housing and inequalities in health: a study of socioeconomic dimensions of housing and self reported health from a survey of Vancouver residents. J Epidemiol Community Health 56(9):671–681, 2002 12177083

Dunn JR, Hayes MV: Identifying social pathways for health inequalities. The role of housing. Ann N Y Acad Sci 896:399–402, 1999 10681934

Elton PJ, Packer JM: A prospective randomised trial of the value of rehousing on the grounds of mental ill-health. J Chronic Dis 39(3):221–227, 1986 3512589

Evans GW: The built environment and mental health. J Urban Health 80(4):536–555, 2003 14709704

Evans GW: Child development and the physical environment. Annu Rev Psychol 57:423–451, 2006 16318602

Evans GW, Lepore SJ, Allen KM: Cross-cultural differences in tolerance for crowding: fact or fiction? J Pers Soc Psychol 79(2):204–210, 2000a 10948974

Evans GW, Wells NM, Chan HY, et al: Housing quality and mental health. J Consult Clin Psychol 68(3):526–530, 2000b 10883571

Evans GW, Wells NM, Moch A: Housing and mental health: a review of the evidence and a methodological and conceptual critique. J Soc Issues 59(3):475–500, 2003

Fazel S, Khosla V, Doll H, et al: The prevalence of mental disorders among the homeless in western countries: systematic review and meta-regression analysis. PLoS Med 5(12):e225, 2008 19053169

Fowler PJ, Henry DB, Schoeny M, et al: Developmental timing of housing mobility: longitudinal effects on externalizing behaviors among at-risk youth. J Am Acad Child Adolesc Psychiatry 53(2):199–208, 2014 24472254

Grant R, Gracy D, Goldsmith G, et al: Twenty-five years of child and family homelessness: where are we now? Am J Public Health 103(Suppl 2):e1–e10, 2013 24148055

Halpern D: Mental Health and the Built Environment. London, Taylor & Francis, 1995

Kenyon C, Sandel M, Silverstein M, et al: Revisiting the social history for child health. Pediatrics 120(3):e734–e738, 2007 17766513

Kessler RC, Duncan GJ, Gennetian LA, et al: Associations of housing mobility interventions for children in high-poverty neighborhoods with subsequent mental disorders during adolescence. JAMA 311(9):937–948, 2014 24595778

Kling J, Liebman J, Klatz L: Experimental analysis of neighborhood effects. Econometrica 75:83–119, 2007

Leventhal T, Newman S: Housing and child development. Child Youth Serv Rev 32:1165–1174, 2010

Magdol L: Is moving gendered? The effects of residential mobility on the psychological well-being of men and women. Sex Roles 47(11–12):553–560, 2002

Matheson FI, Moineddin R, Dunn JR, et al: Urban neighborhoods, chronic stress, gender and depression. Soc Sci Med 63(10):2604–2616, 2006 16920241

Miller KE, Rasmussen A: War exposure, daily stressors, and mental health in conflict and post-conflict settings: bridging the divide between trauma-focused and psychosocial frameworks. Soc Sci Med 70(1):7–16, 2010 19854552

Munoz M, Crespo M, Perez-Santos E: Homeless effects on men's and women's health. J Ment Health 34:47–61, 2005

National Alliance to End Homelessness: The State of Homelessness in America 2013. Washington, DC, National Alliance to End Homelessness, 2013. Available at: http://www.endhomelessness.org/library/entry/the-state-of-homelessness-2013. Accessed April 27, 2014.

National Center for Healthy Housing: State of Healthy Housing. Columbia, MD, National Center for Healthy Housing, 2013. Available at: http://www.nchh.org/Policy/2013StateofHealthyHousing.aspx. Accessed March 6, 2014.

Popkin SJ, Gallagher M, Hailey C, et al: CHA Residents and the Plan for Transformation Long Term Outcomes for CHA Residents. Washington, DC, Urban Institute, 2013. Available at: http://www.urban.org/publications/412761.html. Accessed April 27, 2014.

Reid M, Fiffer M, Gunturi N, et al: Breathe easy at home: a web-based referral system linking clinical sites with housing code enforcement for patients with asthma. J Environ Health 76(7):36–39, 2014 24683937

Rynearson S, Barrett B, Clark C: Housing First: A Review of the Literature. Prepared for the National Center on Homelessness Among Veterans. Tampa, FL, 2010

Sandel M, Wright RJ: When home is where the stress is: expanding the dimensions of housing that influence asthma morbidity. Arch Dis Child 91(11):942–948, 2006 17056870

Shaw M: Housing and public health. Annu Rev Public Health 25:397–418, 2004 15015927

Shenassa ED, Daskalakis C, Liebhaber A, et al: Dampness and mold in the home and depression: an examination of mold-related illness and perceived control of one's home as possible depression pathways. Am J Public Health 97(10):1893–1899, 2007 17761567

Suglia SF, Duarte CS, Sandel MT: Housing quality, housing instability, and maternal mental health. J Urban Health 88(6):1105–1116, 2011 21647798

U.S. Census Bureau: American Housing Survey, 2014. Available at: http://www.census.gov/programs-surveys/ahs. Accessed March 6, 2014.

U.S. Department of Housing and Urban Development: Expanding Housing Choices for HUD-Assisted Families. Washington, DC, U.S. Department of Housing and Urban Development, 1996. Available at: http://www.huduser.org/portal/publications/affhsg/choices.html. Accessed April 27, 2014.

Weich S, Blanchard M, Prince M, et al: Mental health and the built environment: cross-sectional survey of individual and contextual risk factors for depression. Br J Psychiatry 180:428–433, 2002 11983640

Wells NM, Evans GW, Beavis A, et al: Early childhood poverty, cumulative risk exposure, and body mass index trajectories through young adulthood. Am J Public Health 100(12):2507–2512, 2010 20966374

Wood D, Halfon N, Scarlata D, et al: Impact of family relocation on children's growth, development, school function, and behavior. JAMA 270(11):1334–1338, 1993 7689659

Ziol-Guest KM, McKenna CC: Early childhood housing instability and school readiness. Child Dev 85(1):103–113, 2014 23534607

9

Adverse Features of the Built Environment

Lynn C. Todman, Ph.D., M.C.P.

Christopher S. Holliday, Ph.D., M.A., M.P.H.

Where you stand depends on where you sit.

Nelson Mandela, 1918–2013

The built environment is inherently political. It is a reflection of political values and motives, both explicit and implicit. It is encoded with values regarding the living and working conditions merited by different groups of people. It is programmed with motives designed to serve political agendas and to determine who gets access to key resources (e.g., housing) and opportunities (e.g., jobs). Put another way, the built environment is a reflection of the politics governing who thrives in social, economic, and environmental conditions that promote health (including mental health) and who languishes in conditions that compromise health. Thus, the built environment determines health outcomes, including health disparities and inequities. Illuminating the health implications of the built environment is critical to mental health promotion efforts.

The authors wish to acknowledge the helpful feedback provided by Vanessa Salcedo, M.P.H., Research Associate, American Medical Association, and Nikki Bishop, doctoral student at the Adler School of Professional Psychology.

193

In this chapter, we highlight some of the documented relationships between key features of the built environment and mental health and discuss clinical implications of these relationships, including how psychiatrists and other mental health professionals might assess and address the risk factors posed by the built environment. We also present ideas about how mental health providers might use policy interventions, in collaboration with planners, architects, engineers, and others responsible for erecting and managing the built environment, to ensure that the built environment promotes mental health, especially among the most vulnerable.

The Built Environment: An Overview

The built environment is a product of human-driven processes. As a concept, it emerged in the 1980s in the fields of architecture and planning and has since become an important consideration in other disciplines, such as public health. The built environment is characterized by four key attributes: 1) it comprises all things humanly created or modified; 2) its purpose is to serve human needs, wants, and values; 3) it helps humans manage the natural environment to increase comfort and well-being; and 4) it shapes the physical and social environment within which humans function and therefore affects virtually all aspects of human existence and quality of life (McClure and Bartuska 2007).

The built environment is also ubiquitous. It comprises houses, office and school buildings, and stores and factories. It includes the public works infrastructure ranging from roads and bridges to airports and energy-generating facilities. It takes the form of built green space such as landscapes, streetscapes, courtyards, and parks. Significantly, the ubiquity of the built environment renders it "hidden" such that we often fail to recognize it as an important contributor to health. We often fail to appreciate its impacts on human life, including its impacts on mental health.

Adverse Features of the Built Environment as Social Determinants of Health

The built environment has well-documented effects on health—both physical and mental health. Decisions about land use, zoning, and architectural and community design help shape the health determinants to which people are exposed and, as a consequence, their health outcomes. Such decisions determine, for instance, human exposure to environmental toxins; communities' access to public services, amenities, and employment opportunities; and whether a home or neighborhood is safe.

Several examples illustrate the impact of the built environment on physical health. For years, residents of two low-income Latino communities in Chicago experienced high rates of asthma, bronchitis, and emphysema, as well as premature death, because of their physical proximity to highly polluting coal-fired power plants (Environmental Law and Policy Center 2010). Additionally, people who live in *food deserts* (i.e., places that lack easy access to healthy, affordable food) or *food swamps* (i.e., places where unhealthy foods are more readily available than healthy foods) exhibit high rates of obesity, diabetes, and other diet-related conditions and diseases (Ver Ploeg et al. 2009). Studies show that distance from a Level I trauma center is a significant determinant of survival after a gunshot wound (Crandall et al. 2013). Children with close access to parks and recreational resources are less likely to experience significant increases in attained body mass index (Wolch et al. 2011). Social isolation due to poor access to health care, family and friends, and community services and facilities is associated with elevated risk of mortality after a diagnosis of breast cancer (Kroenke et al. 2006). These are just a few of the multitude of ways in which the built environment is known to influence physical health outcomes.

The Built Environment and Mental Health

The built environment also affects mental health and does so in ways that are both direct and indirect. It affects mental health directly through its effects on human auditory, visual, olfactory, and neurological systems. It affects mental health indirectly through its influence on other determinants of mental health, such as social cohesion, social capital, and sense of community.

In this section, we highlight the mental health impacts of four features of the built environment: 1) public works infrastructure (including energy systems, transportation systems, communications systems, and waste management systems), 2) built green space, 3) housing, and 4) schools and workplaces.

Public Works Infrastructure

The public works infrastructure is a massive and multifaceted feature of the built environment. It comprises complex, interactive physical networks, or systems, required to support the economic and social activities that take place in society. Significantly, public works infrastructure is required to ensure the safe, effective, and efficient functioning of other elements of the built environment, such as housing, schools, and office buildings. Four forms of public works infrastructure systems have known mental health impacts, specifically, those pertaining to energy, transportation, communications, and waste management. Some of the components of these systems are given in Table 9–1.

Energy systems are complex and expansive physical networks used to generate, transmit, and distribute electricity or power generated by gas, oil, coal, nuclear fuel, the sun, wind, and water. Energy systems are required for the safe and efficient functioning of virtually all other features of the built environment. They also play important roles in facilitating interactions among people and connecting them to essential goods and services. Thus, energy systems can have tremendous positive and negative impacts on mental health. When they function well, they keep us safe, productive, and socially connected. When they fail, they reduce access to essential supplies such as water and food, undermine safety, and limit social connectedness (Abramson and Redlener 2012).

TABLE 9–1. Some of the components of four forms of public works infrastructure systems

Infrastructure	Components
Energy systems	Physical plants, towers, silos, reactors, conductors, substations, mines, pipelines, wells, refineries, and dams
Transportation systems	Streets and bridges, railroads, airports, water ports, sidewalks, bicycle paths, and walking trails
Communications systems	Numerous forms of physical plants and equipment, including terminals, processors, satellites, and radars
Waste management systems	Landfills, incinerators, storage tanks, and many other facilities and types of equipment

Electricity distribution systems may emit electromagnetic fields, which have been associated with a litany of adverse mental health effects, including anxiety, depression, lethargy, sleeping problems, and Alzheimer's and Parkinson's diseases (Sorahan and Kheifets 2007). In recent years, certain types of energy production, such as mountaintop removal mining and hydraulic fracturing (also known as fracking), have been found to produce negative mental health effects such as depression and anxiety, largely because of the emotional distress asso ciated with destruction of the natural environment and worry about possible physical health effects (Hendryx 2011).

Transportation systems comprise elements of the built environment that facilitate movement of people and goods. Research suggests that transportation systems can affect mental health via two pathways: 1) mobility and accessibility and 2) noise. Road, air, water, and rail systems may influence mental health through their effects on mobility and access to essential goods, services, and employment opportunities, all of which have well-documented mental health impacts. Bicycle paths, sidewalks, and walking trails can have positive mental health effects because they enable mobility and accessibility and also because they encourage physical activity and exercise (Peluso and Guerra de Andrade 2005). Characteristics of street systems, such as traffic-calming cul-de-sacs and road bumps, can positively affect mental health by creating a sense of safety and security. Transportation systems can support mental health by enhancing social and familial networks, social capital, inclusion, and cohesion. On the other hand, problems with transportation systems can harm mental health by blocking or complicating mobility and access required to engage in physical activity, acquire essential goods and services, and participate in social networks. Transportation systems can also harm mental health through the noise they produce. Noise from airports, roads, and rail facilities have been linked to impaired cognition, poorer psychomotor and neurobehavioral performance, and adverse emotional stress responses (van Kempen et al. 2010).

Communications systems are complex networks of sites and facilities required to support human interaction via the telephone, radio, television, and the Internet. Communications systems promote mental health by facilitating access to and functioning of essential goods and services and by supporting social interactions and connections. Although communications systems play an important role in facilitating social connectedness, in modern times some concern has arisen about their potential negative effects on social connections through a process termed *social severance*, which is characterized by an excessive dependence on handheld and other devices (e.g., smartphones) for communication. Additionally, there are concerns regarding the mental health effects of overconnectedness, such as the stress associated with e-mail overload and anxiety associated with Internet-based cyberbullying (Sourander et al. 2010).

Waste management systems include sites and facilities used to transport, destroy, and recycle solid and liquid waste produced in residential, commercial, and industrial settings. The location of waste management facilities is a politically charged issue that often pits communities and municipalities against industries. Community and municipal opposition typically stems from concerns about documented or suspected health effects associated with proximity to such sites, such as cancers and respiratory illnesses, as well as poor maternal health outcomes (Forastiere et al. 2011). Such concerns manifest as stress, fear, and anxiety. Moreover, people living near waste disposal sites have reported a number of psychiatric symptoms, and there is evidence to suggest that people who are exposed to hazardous waste facilities exhibit greater levels of psychiatric morbidity than those who are not (World Health Organization 2007).

Although research has not established definitive causal relationships between waste management systems and mental health, there is credible basis for concern. For instance, many toxins in emissions from incinerators not only are known or suspected carcinogens but also have been implicated in a litany of neurological, mental, behavioral, and social outcomes such as autism, dyslexia, impulsive behavior, attention-deficit/hyperactivity disorder (ADHD), learning difficulties, lowered intelligence, delinquency, violence, depression, Alzheimer's disease, and Parkinson's disease.

This brief review of the literature clearly shows that although the research cannot yet be characterized as indisputable, there is evidence to suggest that public works systems have important mental health implications. Going forward, psychiatrists and other mental health professionals have an important role in conducting additional research that builds on what is currently known about the links between public works infrastructure and mental health.

Built Green Space

Built green space, such as parks, community gardens, courtyards, and streetscapes, have important mental health–enhancing benefits; thus, inadequate green space might be a predictor of poor mental health. Green space can positively affect cognitive functioning and mental health by providing opportunities for social interaction, physical activity, relaxation, and visual and auditory pleasure (Bratman et al. 2012). Research findings on the link between green space and mental health suggest that residents of neighborhoods with high-quality public open spaces are less likely to experience psychosocial distress than residents of neighborhoods with low-quality public open spaces (Francis et al. 2012). Children with ADHD who play regularly in green settings have milder symptoms than children with ADHD who play in built outdoor and indoor settings (Taylor and Ming 2011). Park usage is associated with improved cognition, positive emotions, mental satisfaction and restoration, and improved spiritual health (Irvine et al. 2013). Exposure to parks and gardens is associated with improved cognitive functioning in children and reduced stress in adults (Irvine et al. 2013). Horticulture therapy through active gardening, as well as passive use of gardens, is proven to positively affect mood (Górska-Kłęk et al. 2009). Streetscapes and community gardens can also positively affect mental health by enhancing one's sense of community and increasing social capital (Spokane et al. 2007). Landscapes have the potential to promote mental well-being through attention restoration, stress reduction, and the evocation of positive emotions (Abraham et al. 2010). In summary, natural spaces and built green spaces have mental health–promoting effects, and lack of access to such spaces is likely detrimental to mental health in modern life.

Housing

As described in much greater detail in Chapter 8, "Poor Housing Quality and Housing Instability," numerous investigations have found that housing characterized by poor structural integrity, disrepair, and unpleasant physical attributes is associated with poor mental health. Leaks, draftiness, and dampness; nonfunctioning kitchen appliances, bathroom facilities, and elevators; poor lighting and temperature controls; broken windows and doors; prison-like concrete walls and floors; and building code violations all underlie stress, frustration, anxiety, symptoms of psychological distress, learned helplessness, and lower task persistence (Turney et al. 2013). Other linkages between housing and mental health are shown in Table 9–2 (Evans 2003; McFarlane et al. 2013).

Schools and Workplaces

For most children and adults, the majority of waking hours are spent either in school or at a place of work. Therefore, the design, layout, and

TABLE 9–2. Examples of associations between housing conditions and poor mental health outcomes

Housing conditions	Mental health outcomes
Housing characterized by poor structural integrity, disrepair, and unpleasant physical attributes	Poor mental health
Living on the upper floors of high-rise apartment buildings	Psychological distress
Small-scale residential facilities that are quiet and that accommodate wandering	Improved functioning in individuals with Alzheimer's disease
High residential density and overcrowding	Behavioral problems in children
Poor indoor air quality and ambient toxins	Negative affect
Insufficient daylight	Symptoms of depression
Exposure to lead in paint, dust, soil, and drinking water	Mental and behavioral conditions, including brain and neurological damage that leads to emotional, behavioral, and learning problems, as well as low intelligence quotient (IQ) and several neurological disorders

physical characteristics of these spaces have the potential to significantly affect mental health. There is strong, consistent evidence that the built school environment—from single-building structures to large campuses with multiple classrooms, common areas, lunchrooms, sports fields, and offices—has an impact on children's behavioral health. For instance, poor-quality school buildings have been associated with vandalism, absenteeism, suspensions, disciplinary incidents, violence, and smoking among students (Schneider 2002). Chronic noise endured by children in schools located near airports adversely affects cognitive functioning and increases irritability and psychological stress (van Kempen et al. 2010). Noise in open-plan schools with few floor-to-ceiling walls is similarly problematic (Anderson 2001). However, these open-plan schools may support positive mental health by offering opportunities for social inter-action, cohesion, and bonding (Gislason 2009), which exemplifies the complexity inherent in considering the built environment.

The distance from children's homes to schools can amplify a sense of loneliness and anxiety, adversely affect children's personal and social well-being, and decrease their sense of community and personal con-nection to their surroundings (Jackson and Tester 2008). The location of schools outside of neighborhoods in which children live can also adversely affect their mental health if their commute is long, compli-cated, and/or involves crossing gang lines and other social barriers (Ahmed-Ullah and Nix 2013).

School buildings with natural light through windows and skylights are associated with more positive mood and mental outlook (Mead 2008). Chil-dren in windowless classrooms have been shown to experience distur-bances in diurnal cortisol rhythms and concentration compared with children in classrooms with windows (Kuller and Lindsten 1992). Artificial light, such as incandescent and fluorescent lights found in some class-rooms, has been shown to induce stress, aggression, irritability, and hyper-activity and to reduce concentration (Human Ecological Social Economic Project 2013). Although the evidence is conflicting, scholars have noted that wall and decor color can affect mood and mental clarity as well as produc-tivity, concentration, and accuracy (Yildirim et al. 2007). Additionally, class-rooms that are dense and overcrowded have been shown to decrease academic performance and increase behavioral problems (Maxwell 2003).

Temperature, heating, and air quality have documented impacts on students' behavior and achievement (Lemasters and Earthman 2011). Additionally, poor indoor climatic conditions due to, for instance, ill-maintained ventilation or poor air conditioning systems may affect lev-els of carbon monoxide and thereby adversely influence students' mental health and academic performance (Schneider 2002). Physical organiza-tion of classrooms also has an impact on behavior (Higgins et al. 2005).

Built forms, such as school playgrounds with vegetation, school-administered gardens, and parks, play important roles in children's mental health and emotional well-being by reducing aggression and stress; improving cognition, positive emotions, mental satisfaction, restoration, and spiritual health; reducing ADHD symptoms; and encouraging play and social integration (Jackson and Tester 2008; Taylor and Ming 2011).

There is ample evidence to suggest that the workplace environment also has both direct and indirect effects on adults' mental health and well-being. For instance, workplace design can affect mental health via the effects of office light exposure on circadian regulation, social behavior, and affect; the effects of office aesthetics on mood; access to nature and recovery from stressful experiences; and privacy regulation and stimulus control (Veitch 2011). Office views that are more attractive and include natural elements reduce stress and discomfort at work, induce better sleep quality at home, increase life satisfaction, and increase attentional capacity (Aries et al. 2010; Bratman et al. 2012). Natural elements in the built health care environment, such as indoor plants, also have been shown to reduce stress levels (Dijkstra et al. 2008).

Documented mental and behavioral health effects (e.g., stress, frustration, and impaired attention) are associated with spatial density, ceiling height, and open-plan cubicles versus private offices that allow better control over noise and temperature (Jahncke et al. 2011; Veitch 2011). Sick building syndrome (i.e., a group of symptoms attributed to the physical environment of specific buildings) can be due to poorly functioning heating, ventilation, and air-conditioning systems (Crawford and Bolas 1996). Office heating and cooling systems may also have an impact on mental health (e.g., workers' comfort, stress levels, and task accuracy) through thermal comfort, which is a function of the right combination of temperature, airflow, and humidity (Tanabe et al. 2007).

Adverse Features of the Built Environment in the Clinical Setting

Case Example: Emergency Department Patients in the Westwood Community

Dr. Scott Chapman is an emergency medicine physician. He recently began working at Westwood Community Hospital, which is located in a low-income neighborhood of a small Rust Belt town. At the hospital, Dr. Chapman provides care for many Medicaid and Medicare beneficiaries and some uninsured patients. In his brief time at the hospital to date, Dr. Chapman has noticed that the emergency department (ED) has a high number of patients with mental and neurological disorders. For instance, in a recent 10-hour shift, he encountered the following patients.

Tiffany Williams, a 12-year-old girl, presented with a severe asthma exacerbation. Her mother, Yvonne Williams, 32 years old, brought Tiffany to the ED and explained that in recent months, Tiffany's teachers have complained of behavioral problems. In addition, Tiffany has recently exhibited signs of depression.

Dr. Chapman also evaluated Ms. Williams herself. She has diabetes and indicated that she has been having problems with focus, lethargy, and sleep. Ms. Williams spoke of one bright spot in her life: she recently got a job at the new power plant. Unfortunately, because she works long hours cleaning the facility at night, she is not able to spend much time with Tiffany. Ms. Williams indicated that both her and Tiffany's conditions seem to have worsened since she started the new job. Dr. Chapman referred both Tiffany and her mother to Dr. Dolores Rivera, the on-call psychiatrist. Dr. Rivera met with them and determined that although Tiffany is safe for now, a follow-up at her school's health center is indicated. Dr. Rivera also scheduled a follow-up appointment for Ms. Williams.

During his shift, Dr. Chapman also cared for Francisco Fernandez, a 55-year-old father of three. He was brought in by his wife, who stated that Mr. Fernandez had lost his job of 20 years when an old manufacturing facility was shuttered. Since then, he has had difficulty with concentration and memory and has been spending a considerable amount of time in bed. His wife is also concerned because she has noticed that he has recently increased his drinking substantially. Again, Dr. Chapman paged Dr. Rivera, who determined that Mr. Fernandez exhibited signs and symptoms of anxiety, depression, and alcohol misuse.

Subsequently, Dr. Chapman examined Joseph Turner, a 62-year-old man with early signs of Parkinson's disease. Mr. Turner reported developing a tremor at the beginning of the year that appears to have worsened in recent months. He also seemed depressed. A call to Dr. Rivera was, again, the next order of business.

Finally, Dr. Chapman evaluated 26-year-old Peter Kim, who presented with a knife wound but also complained of hearing voices and feeling in danger because he felt that he was being spied on through the television. He also revealed that a long list of people were "out to get" him. His girlfriend, Aida, shared that sometimes he experiences periods of confusion or detachment that seem to occur unexpectedly and are not clearly related to his concurrent marijuana use. Both Dr. Chapman and Dr. Rivera tried to engage Mr. Kim, but he indicated that he did not trust either of them.

As Dr. Chapman reflects on the many patients he has seen since the beginning of his tenure at the hospital who presented with diagnosed or suspected mental, substance use, and neurological problems, he wonders, "What are the underlying causes resulting in so many people in a small community having such challenges?" Might they share some hidden risk factors that he was not aware of or attending to in the ED?

Assessing Adverse Features of the Built Environment in the Clinical Setting

Numerous factors likely underlie the high rates of behavioral and neurological problems among ED patients of the Westwood Community Hospital. To discover what they might be, it would be instructive to ask questions about what these patients have in common. If we consider the possible role of the built environment, we might ask the following:

What are their neighborhoods like? Are the streets well lit, and therefore, do they evoke a sense of safety and security? Are there available parks and open spaces for recreation and relaxation? Are the neighborhoods physically remote in a way that brings about social isolation? Or are they located near a range of transit options that facilitate access to essential goods, services, and amenities? Are the neighborhoods located near heavy industry or any other sources of air, land, or noise pollution? What is the housing like? Is it well maintained, up to code, and structurally sound? If employed, where do people work? Do they have access to natural sunlight during the daytime? What are the schools like? Are they overcrowded? Do children have outdoor spaces in which to play and interact? Are workplaces and schools within reasonable commuting distances? Taken together, how might the built environment affect the health of Dr. Chapman's community?

Typically, neither emergency physicians nor psychiatrists and other mental health professionals ask these types of questions. However, such queries are important because there are documented mental health implications of public works systems, green space, housing structures, school buildings, and workplaces. Following this line of inquiry, Dr. Chapman discovered that most of the patients he sees live in a large public housing complex that suffers from deferred maintenance (e.g., broken windows, intermittently working heating and cooling systems, and poorly functioning kitchen facilities) and numerous building code violations (e.g., lead paint and pipes). The disrepair invites criminal activity that evokes fear, stress, and anxiety in the residents and undermines their sense of safety and security. The complex is also downwind from the new coal-fired power plant, built a year ago after a highly charged and politicized public debate about its location. Residents of affluent communities were able to effectively quash proposals that the facility be located near them, despite the large swaths of available land. The lack of social cohesion among Westwood's public housing residents, and thus lack of community activism, served as an opening for locating the facility near their community. Although the new jobs are beneficial and the local transportation system would not have supported commutes from Westwood to other proposed sites for the facility, now that the plant is at full capacity, it is noisy, especially at night, and it emits waste materials into the air and the adjacent waterway, causing insomnia and anxiety about air and water pollution.

In addition to being in disrepair, the housing complex is visually menacing—a graffiti-marked, concrete, multistory edifice that does not have nearby green or open spaces for relaxation, recreation, and social activities. The lack of community gathering spaces means that there is little opportunity for engagement among residents, and as a result, many residents feel socially disconnected and isolated.

Dr. Chapman also discovers that as a result of a shrinking tax base (shuttered factories and failing small businesses), severe budget constraints, the steady depopulation of the region, and the recent closures of increasingly underpopulated schools, the neighborhood school that Tiffany had attended since kindergarten was recently closed. The school she now attends is 30 miles away from her home and not easily or efficiently accessible via public transit, which is the mode of transportation most heavily relied on by residents of her public housing complex. Ms. Williams does not have a car, and even if she did, she would be hard-pressed to take Tiffany to school after her night shift at the plant. After taking two buses, Tiffany must walk the last half mile to get to her new school, adding an extra hour to her morning and afternoon commutes. Like her mother, she does not get enough sleep.

How Clinicians Can Address Adverse Features of the Built Environment

Given the large numbers of people who present to the ED with mental health problems, in addition to treating the symptoms presented by each individual with psychotropic medications and behavioral interventions, Drs. Chapman and Rivera can also seek solutions to the broader social determinants of their patients' health, including aspects of the built environment in which their patients live and work. In doing so, Dr. Chapman discovers that his patients are vulnerable to living and working conditions—shaped by the built environment—that research suggests predispose people to behavioral and neurological disorders. Psychiatrists and other mental health professionals can produce better physical and mental health outcomes by being advocates for their patients. Doing so may require working with planners, architects, civil engineers, and others who are responsible for planning, creating, and maintaining the built environment. In addition, and perhaps more importantly, clinicians can serve as patient advocates in local, state, and federal policy discussions. In both instances, their work can help ensure that the environment to which their patients are exposed promotes good mental health and well-being.

Policy Approaches to Adverse Features of the Built Environment

As noted earlier, the political context that shapes the built environment is not value neutral. The political context reflects a very specific set of cultural values, norms, and beliefs about the allocation of resources, rights, and opportunities among different communities and population subgroups. Those values, norms, and beliefs (i.e., who is deserving of governmental support and who is not, what constitutes legitimate support and what does not, and relative commitment to personal responsibility compared with social responsibility) are reflected in public policy. That policy, with all its encoded values and beliefs, shapes the social determinants of mental health, including the built environment. Thus, policy plays a very powerful role in shaping mental health outcomes; it can (and does) ensure optimal mental health for some communities, and it can (and does) yield suboptimal mental health for others. Over time, therefore, policies may create and sustain health disparities and inequities.

Health in All Policies and the Built Environment

By engaging in policy-making processes, psychiatrists and other mental health professionals can play an important "nonclinical" role in shaping health outcomes that manifest in clinical settings. For instance, they can engage in land use policy development to help ensure that families do not live near industrial or commercial facilities that pose health threats due to air, land, water, or noise pollution. They can help craft planning policies to ensure that all people have access to health-enhancing open and green space. They can help facilitate the development and enforcement of housing policy to ensure that homes are structurally sound, free of toxic materials, and adherent to mandated building codes. They can work to ensure that transportation policy provides multiple, convenient transit options giving everyone access to services, goods, and amenities required for good health. They can work on occupational safety and education legislation to ensure that workplaces and schools afford opportunities for exposure to natural light and space for social interaction and have indoor temperatures, air quality, and physical layouts that support good mental health. They can work on fiscal and economic policy to ensure that social welfare supports are well funded and that their patients have living wages that allow them to have access to quality housing, education, and nutritious food and other requisites to good health. How might they do this? One way is by joining the Health in All Policies (HiAP) movement (Commission on Social Determinants of Health 2008).

HiAP is a growing national and international effort to increase policy makers' and citizens' understanding of the health consequences of policy decisions. HiAP reflects a growing understanding that public policies of all types (e.g., those pertaining to energy, land use, the environment, housing, transportation, employment, food, and education) have health implications. In fact, a growing theme within the movement states that "all policies are health policies." There is a case to be made that all policies are also mental health policies. Practically, how can psychiatrists and other mental health professionals join this movement? One way is by participating in Health Impact Assessments (HIAs) and Mental Health Impact Assessments (MHIAs). Another way is by engaging in advocacy work on behalf of their patients and the communities where both they and their patients live, go to school, work, and play.

HIAs are a practice increasingly used by public health professionals, policy makers, and entire communities worldwide to help ensure that public policy affects social conditions in ways that promote health. MHIAs, pioneered by the Center for the Social Determinants of Mental Health at the Adler School of Professional Psychology, are used to help ensure that policy decisions promote mental health as well (Todman et al. 2012).

HIAs and MHIAs involve a six-step process in which scientific data and community opinion are used to prospectively assess the health impacts of a policy (or legislative, planning, programmatic, or project proposal) on the health of a population. Intended to be a preventive practice, the results of HIAs and MHIAs are used to develop interventions that enhance any protective features and mitigate any health risks that the policy or proposal might create or exacerbate. Significantly, HIAs and MHIAs provide information that serves as the basis for health advocacy.

Mental Health Professionals as Community Health Advocates

Psychiatrists and other mental health professionals can join the HiAP movement by engaging in advocacy work such as collaborations with people and organizations seeking to combat structural and systematic inequities that harm health. There is a long and rich history of physician advocates who have played important roles in improving the social conditions that have an impact on health. Jackson and Tester (2008) noted that during the twentieth century, for instance, physicians, as daily witnesses to the ill health caused by contaminated water and intense crowding, were valuable advocates in the efforts to improve people's living environments. The role of the physician is just as critical today: the challenges are different, but the environment still shapes many of our health problems, including those of mental health. (p. 129)

In the early years of the twenty-first century, the need for physicians as advocates continues. Consider the American Medical Association's *Declaration of Professional Responsibility*, which includes the following: "Advocate for social, economic, educational, and political changes that ameliorate suffering and contribute to human well-being" (American Medical Association 2001). Physician commitment to this declaration was demonstrated in a 2006 study published in the *Journal of the American Medical Association* in which a majority of the 1,662 physicians surveyed rated community participation and collective advocacy as "very important" (Gruen et al. 2006).

Physicians can engage in advocacy through a number of avenues. Programs such as the Physicians as Community Health Advocates leadership program work to prepare physicians for advocacy and other leadership roles in the communities they serve so that they can help advance policies and other public decisions that promote health (American Medical Association 2014). The Institute on Medicine as a Profession (2011) has developed a Physician Advocacy Program and a Physician Advocacy Fellowship, both of which support and encourage doctors to use their experience and expertise to advocate for the policy changes required to ensure that social determinants of health, such as those associated with the built environment, have a positive impact on health outcomes.

Promoting a Built Environment That Supports Mental Health: A Role for Everyone

Given the documented and suspected relationships between the built environment and mental health, it is incumbent on psychiatrists and other mental health professionals to collaborate with planners, architects, civil engineers, and others who are responsible for designing, erecting, managing, and maintaining the built environment to ensure that it promotes mental health. To this end, transdisciplinary research and collaborations will be critical going forward. Psychiatrists and other mental health professionals must participate in scholarly efforts to better understand how the massive public works systems that comprise an enormous amount of the nation's built form affect mental health, how school and workplace designs affect emotional and cognitive functioning, and how living near heavy industry or chronic noise emitters affects psychological well-being. Equally important, there is an urgent need for mental health professionals to actively engage in translating existing and emerging knowledge and insights into policy and practice.

Key Points

- The built environment is inherently political, with powerful implications for mental health outcomes, including mental health disparities and inequities.

- The built environment is ubiquitous, subtle, and often "invisible," with the result that it affects mental health in ways that are often overlooked and therefore unaddressed.

- The built environment affects mental health in ways that are both direct and indirect. Its impacts are, at times, explicitly evident; at other times, they must be inferred through their effects on physical health and on other social determinants (e.g., social capital and cohesion) that are known to have mental health implications.

- To promote mental health, especially that of the most vulnerable citizens, clinicians must use what is currently understood about the relationship between the built environment and mental health to influence policy pertaining to the built environment.

- Clinicians must engage in transdisciplinary work, including both research and practice, with professionals in other fields such as planning, architecture, and civil engineering to continue inquiry into and advance discovery with regard to the relationship between the built environment and mental health.

References

Abraham A, Sommerhalder K, Abel T: Landscape and well-being: a scoping study on the health-promoting impact of outdoor environments. Int J Public Health 55(1):59 69, 2010 19768384

Abramson DM, Redlener I: Hurricane Sandy: lessons learned, again. Disaster Med Public Health Prep 6(4):328–329, 2012 23241461

Ahmed-Ullah N, Nix N: CPS sets Safe Passage routes: parents remain wary as they send kids across gang lines. Chicago Tribune, August 9, 2013

Anderson K: Kids in noisy classrooms: what does the research really say? Journal of Educational Audiology 9:21–33, 2001

American Medical Association: Declaration of Professional Responsibility: Medicine's Social Contract With Humanity. Chicago, IL, American Medical Association, 2001

American Medical Association: Community Health Leadership. Chicago, IL, American Medical Association, 2014. Available at: http://www.ama-assn.org/ama/pub/physician-resources/public-health/promoting-healthy-lifestyles/community-health-leadership.page?. Accessed April 16, 2014.

Aries M, Veitch J, Newsham GR: Windows, view, and office characteristics predict physical and psychological discomfort. J Environ Psychol 30(4):533–541, 2010

Bratman GN, Hamilton JP, Daily GC: The impacts of nature experience on human cognitive function and mental health. Ann N Y Acad Sci 1249:118–136, 2012 22320203

Commission on Social Determinants of Health: Closing the Gap in a Generation: Health Equity Through Action on the Social Determinants of Health. Final Report of the Commission on Social Determinants of Health. Geneva, World Health Organization, 2008

Crandall M, Sharp D, Unger E, et al: Trauma deserts: distance from a trauma center, transport times, and mortality from gunshot wounds in Chicago. Am J Public Health 103(6):1103–1109, 2013 23597339

Crawford JO, Bolas SM: Sick building syndrome, work factors and occupational stress. Scand J Work Environ Health 22(4):243–250, 1996 8881012

Dijkstra K, Pieterse ME, Pruyn A: Stress-reducing effects of indoor plants in the built healthcare environment: the mediating role of perceived attractiveness. Prev Med 47(3):279–283, 2008 18329704

Environmental Law and Policy Center: Midwest Generation's "Unpaid Health Bills": The Hidden Public Costs of Soot and Smog From the Fisk and Crawford Coal Plants in Chicago. Chicago, IL, Environmental Law and Policy Center, 2010. Available at: http://elpc.org/wp-content/uploads/2010/10/MidwestGenerationsUnpaidHealthBillsFormattedFinal.pdf. Accessed February 19, 2014.

Evans GW: The built environment and mental health. J Urban Health 80(4):536–555, 2003 14709704

Forastiere F, Badaloni C, de Hoogh K, et al: Health impact assessment of waste management facilities in three European countries. Environ Health 10:53, 2011 21635784

Francis J, Wood LJ, Knuiman M, et al: Quality or quantity? Exploring the relationship between public open space attributes and mental health in Perth, Western Australia. Soc Sci Med 74(10):1570–1577, 2012 22464220

Gislason N: Mapping school design: a qualitative study of the relations among facilities design, curriculum delivery, and school climate. J Environ Educ 40(4):17–33, 2009

Górska-Kłęk L, Adamczyk K, Sobiech K: Hortitherapy—complementary method in physiotherapy. Physiotherapy 17(4):71–77, 2009

Gruen RL, Campbell EG, Blumenthal D: Public roles of US physicians: community participation, political involvement, and collective advocacy. JAMA 296(20):2467–2475, 2006 17119143

Hendryx M: Poverty and mortality disparities in central Appalachia: mountaintop mining and environmental justice. J Health Dispar Res Pract 4(3):44–53, 2011

Higgins S, Hall E, Wall K, et al: The impact of school environments: a literature review. London, The Centre for Learning and Teaching School of Education, Communication and Language Science, University of Newcastle, The Design Council, 2005. Available at: http://www.ncl.ac.uk/cflat/news/DCReport.pdf. Accessed October 1, 2014.

Human Ecological Social Economic Project: Artificial Light in the Environment: Human Health Effects. Rotenburg, Germany, H.E.S.E. Project, 2013. Available at: http://www.hese-project.org/hese-uk/en/issues/cfl.php. Accessed January 11, 2014.

Institute on Medicine as a Profession: Physician Advocacy Program Overview. New York, Institute on Medicine as a Profession, 2011. http://imapny.org/physician-advocacy/physician-advocacy-program-overview. Accessed November 7, 2013.

Irvine KN, Warber SL, Devine-Wrigth P, et al: Understanding urban green space as a health resource: a qualitative comparison of visit motivation and derived effects among park users in Sheffield, UK. Int J Environ Res Pub Health 10(1):417–442, 2013

Jackson RJ, Tester J: Environment shapes health, including children's mental health. J Am Acad Child Adolesc Psychiatry 47(2):129–131, 2008 18216714

Jahncke H, Hygge S, Halin N, et al: Open-plan office noise: cognitive performance and restoration. J Environ Psychol 31(4):373–382, 2011

Kroenke CH, Kubzansky LD, Schernhammer ES, et al: Social networks, social support, and survival after breast cancer diagnosis. J Clin Oncol 24(7):1105–1111, 2006 16505430

Kuller R, Lindsten C: Health and behavior of children in classrooms with and without windows. J Environ Psychol 12(4):305–317, 1992

Lemasters L, Earthman G: Study of the Relationship Between Air-Conditioned Classrooms and Student Achievement. Scottsdale, AZ, Council of Educational Facilities Planner International, 2011. Available at: http://www.cefpi.org/i4a/ams/amsstore/category.cfm?product_id=115. Accessed April 28, 2014.

Maxwell L: Home and school density effects on elementary school children: the role of spatial density. Environ Behav 4:566–578, 2003

McClure WR, Bartuska TJ: The Built Environment: A Collaborative Inquiry Into Design and Planning. Hoboken, NJ, Wiley, 2007

McFarlane AC, Searle AK, Van Hooff M, et al: Prospective associations between childhood low-level lead exposure and adult mental health problems: the Port Pirie cohort study. Neurotoxicology 39:11–17, 2013 23958641

Mead MN: Benefits of sunlight: a bright spot for human health. Environ Health Perspect 116(4):A160–A167, 2008 18414615

Peluso MA, Guerra de Andrade LH: Physical activity and mental health: the association between exercise and mood. Clinics (Sao Paulo) 60(1):61–70, 2005 15838583

Schneider M: Do School Facilities Affect Academic Outcomes? Washington, DC, National Clearinghouse for Educational Facilities, 2002. Available at: http://www.mphaweb.org/documents/DoSchoolFacilitiesAffectAcademic Outcomes.pdf. Accessed April 28, 2014.

Sorahan T, Kheifets L: Mortality from Alzheimer's, motor neuron and Parkinson's disease in relation to magnetic field exposure: findings from the study of UK electricity generation and transmission workers, 1973–2004. Occup Environ Med 64(12):820–826, 2007 17626136

Sourander A, Brunstein Klomek A, Ikonen M, et al: Psychosocial risk factors associated with cyberbullying among adolescents: a population-based study. Arch Gen Psychiatry 67(7):720–728, 2010 20603453

Spokane AR, Lombard JL, Martinez F, et al: Identifying streetscape features significant to well-being. Archit Sci Rev 50(3):234–245, 2007 23144498

Tanabe S, Nishihara N, Haneda M: Indoor temperature, productivity, and fatigue in office tasks. HVAC&R Research 13:623–633, 2007

Taylor A, Ming F: Could exposure to everyday green spaces help treat ADHD? Evidence from children's play settings. Applied Psychology: Health and Well-Being 3:281–303, 2011

Todman L, Hricisak L, Fay J, et al: Mental health impact assessment: population mental health in Englewood, Chicago, Illinois, USA. Impact Assessment and Project Appraisal 30(2):116–123, 2012

Turney K, Kissane R, Edin K: After Moving to Opportunity: how moving to a low-poverty neighborhood improves mental health among African American women. Society and Mental Health 3(1):1–21, 2013

van Kempen E, van Kamp I, Lebret E, et al: Neurobehavioral effects of transportation noise in primary schoolchildren: a cross-sectional study. Environ Health 9:25, 2010 20515466

Veitch JA: Workplace design contributions to mental health and well-being. Healthc Pap 11(spec no):38–46, 2011 24917255

Ver Ploeg M, Breneman V, Farrigan T, et al: Access to Affordable and Nutritious Food: Measuring and Understanding Food Deserts and Their Consequences. Report to Congress (Administrative Publication No [AP-036]). Washington, DC, U.S. Department of Agriculture, Economic Research Service, 2009

Wolch J, Jerrett M, Reynolds K, et al: Childhood obesity and proximity to urban parks and recreational resources: a longitudinal cohort study. Health Place 17(1):207–214, 2011 21075670

World Health Organization: Population Health and Waste Management: Scientific Data and Policy Options. Report of a WHO Workshop. Copenhagen, World Heath Organization. Available at: http://www.euro.who.int/__data/assets/pdf_file/0012/91101/E91021.pdf. Accessed on October 22, 2013.

Yildirim K, Akalinbaskaya A, Hidayetoglu M: Effects of indoor color on mood and cognitive performance. Building and Environment 42(9):3233–3240, 2007

10

Poor Access to Health Care

Frederick J. P. Langheim, M.D., Ph.D.
Ruth S. Shim, M.D., M.P.H.
Benjamin G. Druss, M.D., M.P.H.

*Of all the forms of inequality, injustice in health
care is the most shocking and inhumane.*

Martin Luther King Jr., 1929–1968

The health care delivery system in the United States is an important factor in determining American citizens' health and well-being. Similarly, the health care delivery system has a major impact on the effective treatment and management of mental illnesses and substance use disorders. The Substance Abuse and Mental Health Services Administration estimated that nearly 46 million U.S. adults had mental illnesses in 2010 (Substance Abuse and Mental Health Services Administration 2012b). Total expenditures in 2005 for mental health treatment and substance abuse treatment in the United States were $113 billion and $22 billion, respectively (Mark et al. 2011). Mental illnesses and substance use disorders are expensive, even without factoring in disability or workplace costs due to lost productivity (Greenberg et al. 2003). However, only 39.2% of adults experiencing a mental illness in 2010 received any type of mental health care. The health care system is a social determinant of health (i.e., it is constructed by us, and it is under our control rather than being genetic/predetermined), and it interacts with and is affected by the other social determinants of health (World Health Organization 2008). Access to quality mental health care in the United States is a major challenge and a social factor that can contribute to a person's mental health and wellness (U.S. Department of Health and Human Services 2013). Insurance coverage—more specifically, adequate mental health coverage—undoubtedly plays a major role in accessing quality mental health services. Although insurance coverage is anticipated to significantly increase under the Affordable Care Act (ACA), gaps in health care coverage will continue to exist because a portion of the U.S. population will remain uninsured.

Unfortunately, insurance coverage alone does not guarantee access to services. Various interconnected factors contribute to poor access to mental health and substance abuse treatment services, and these factors must be addressed at multiple levels to ensure that individuals with behavioral health problems are able to appropriately access care. At the individual level, a person with a mental illness or substance use disorder must recognize and accept the presence of a problem in order to seek or be directed to mental health treatment. Self-stigma, or internalization of stigmatizing attitudes of the public, interferes with treatment engagement and contributes to an individual's choice not to access needed mental health services (Corrigan 2004). To effectively access care, individuals must also address barriers in transportation, financial strain, difficulties with missing work for appointments, and managing the many other competing priorities in modern life.

From a provider's perspective, clinicians must be available to readily evaluate and treat patients in a timely manner and must continuously address scheduling, customer service, quality, and performance improvement issues. Providers must build rapport and therapeutic alliances with patients in order to engage them in ongoing treatment. Furthermore, workforce shortages are a significant driver of problems related to accessing mental health services (Hoge et al. 2009). Primary care providers often have as much difficulty as patients in attempting to access specialty mental health services for their patients, citing mental health workforce shortages, uninsurance or underinsurance, and health plan barriers as major obstacles in their ability to refer patients to mental health services (Cunningham 2009).

From a systems-level perspective, public stigma, lack of insurance, underinsurance, lack of mental health parity, fragmentation of services, and inequalities within funding of the public mental health system all contribute to massive challenges for persons attempting to navigate the mental health system. Also, as a result of the patient-, provider-, and systems-level challenges in accessing mental health services, certain populations are more likely to be susceptible to poor access to mental health care, contributing to worsening mental health inequalities among certain racial/ethnic minority groups as well as geographically isolated populations.

Together, these barriers dramatically lower the likelihood of accessing mental health services because all factors, across individual, provider, and systems levels, must be aligned for an individual to successfully access mental health services. Unfortunately, the threats to accessing care often return with each subsequent follow-up visit (Figure 10–1).

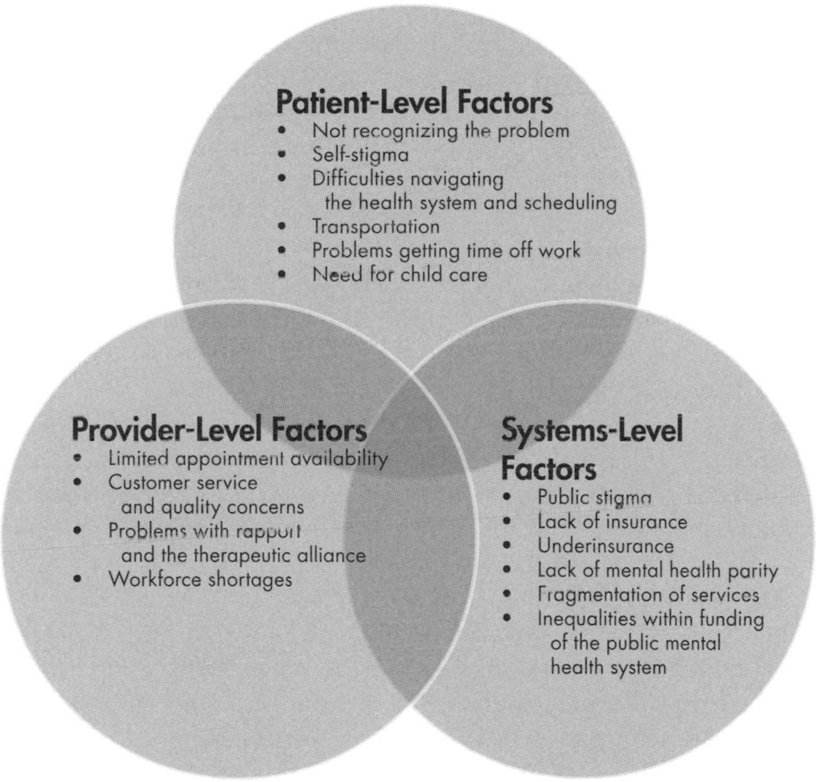

Patient-Level Factors
- Not recognizing the problem
- Self-stigma
- Difficulties navigating the health system and scheduling
- Transportation
- Problems getting time off work
- Need for child care

Provider-Level Factors
- Limited appointment availability
- Customer service and quality concerns
- Problems with rapport and the therapeutic alliance
- Workforce shortages

Systems-Level Factors
- Public stigma
- Lack of insurance
- Underinsurance
- Lack of mental health parity
- Fragmentation of services
- Inequalities within funding of the public mental health system

FIGURE 10–1. Some of the diverse barriers to accessing mental health services.

Defining and Quantifying Poor Access to Care

Access to health care is defined by the Institute of Medicine as "the timely use of personal health services to achieve the best possible health outcomes" (Millman 1993, p. 4). In contrast, poor access to health care encompasses all of the barriers that exist within the system that contribute to individuals' difficulty receiving quality health care services. Although there are significant challenges to accessing appropriate health care services in the United States, access to high-quality mental health care is an even greater multifaceted challenge.

Lack of Insurance Coverage

The U.S. Census Bureau estimated that almost 48 million people were without health insurance in 2012, which is approximately 15% of the U.S. population (U.S. Census Bureau 2013). Lack of health insurance is associated with receiving less preventive care, having more undiagnosed chronic conditions, and experiencing poorer health outcomes (Ayanian et al. 2000, 2003; Institute of Medicine 2002). More specifically, insurance coverage is strongly related to mental health service utilization in that insured individuals are more likely to seek and receive mental health treatment than those who are uninsured (Landerman et al. 1994). With respect to serious mental illnesses such as schizophrenia, major depressive disorder, and bipolar disorder, 20% of individuals with these diagnoses are uninsured (McAlpine and Mechanic 2000). The current health insurance coverage model in the United States is predominantly employment based, and individuals with serious mental illnesses often have high levels of disability, unemployment, or underemployment that can prohibit them from entering the private, employment-based health insurance market (Koyanagi and Siegwarth 2010).

Rates of being uninsured are significantly higher in specific population groups. For example, African Americans and Hispanics are less likely to have insurance coverage than whites, are more likely to have public insurance than private insurance, and are more likely to be enrolled in low-quality health care plans that impose strict limitations on coverage (Smedley et al. 2009). Similarly, individuals living in poverty are significantly less likely to have health insurance than individuals and families with greater household income (DeNavas-Walt et al. 2010). Geographic variation also exists for insurance coverage. Individuals in the South are more likely to be uninsured than those in other regions of the country, and foreign-born citizens are more likely to be uninsured than native-born citizens in the United States (U.S. Census Bureau 2013). Accessing health care is even more problematic for undocumented immigrant populations.

Inequalities in Mental Health Insurance Coverage and Mental Health Parity

Among those with insurance, mental health insurance coverage may be inadequate, and it is often complex to navigate. A patient may have high deductibles that result in self-rationing of behavioral health services. The number of high-deductible insurance plans has increased considerably over the past decade. In 2006, only 10% of plans had deductibles greater than $1,000 for individuals and $2,000 for families. The number of high-deductible plans increased to 22% by 2009 (Claxton et al. 2009). Similarly, because public-sector insurance often provides health care coverage to individuals of lower socioeconomic status, patients with Medicaid may face competing economic priorities that make it difficult to afford co-pays and other expenses associated with mental health treatment (Briesacher et al. 2010).

Even with insurance, mental health coverage is not guaranteed. In the past, and to a lesser extent still today, unequal benefits for mental illnesses when compared with those for physical illnesses have threatened the ability of insured individuals to access appropriate and affordable mental health services. These inequalities have included capping annual and lifetime benefits for mental health care, limits on hospital days and numbers of office visits compared with those for general medical conditions, and higher levels of coinsurance or other cost sharing (Mechanic and McAlpine 1999). Several recent advances have moved toward greater equality between mental health and physical health insurance coverages, including the passage of the Paul Wellstone and Pete Domenici Mental Health Parity and Addiction Equity Act (MHPAEA) in 2008, the recent institution of the "final rule" that determines the effective implementation of the MHPAEA, and the ACA.

Mental Health Workforce Shortages

Difficulties in accessing mental health services are not limited to insurance coverage issues. For a number of reasons, even with high-quality insurance, accessing a timely intake evaluation may be extremely challenging. This difficulty was demonstrated in a study in which researchers posing as psychiatric patients insured by Blue Cross Blue

Shield of Massachusetts contacted all of the mental health facilities within 10 miles of downtown Boston, reporting that they had been evaluated in an emergency department and were instructed to follow up with a psychiatrist within 2 weeks. Of 64 facilities contacted, only 8 (12.5%) offered appointments. In addition, just 4 (6.2%) offered an appointment within the recommended 2-week time period. Underscoring the barriers to care, approximately 23% of phone calls were never returned (Boyd et al. 2011). Furthermore, in some areas it is common for psychiatrists and psychologists to not accept insurance (i.e., cash-only private or group practices) because of low insurance reimbursement rates.

Previous research has estimated that workforce needs vary by geographic region, but methodological challenges make it difficult to precisely measure workforce shortages. Recent estimates have suggested that approximately 25 psychiatrists per 100,000 adult population are needed to adequately address the mental health needs of the U.S. population (Konrad et al. 2009). Unfortunately, the number of practicing psychiatrists falls significantly below this goal: it is estimated that there were 16.5 psychiatrists per 100,000 members of the U.S. population in 2000 (Scully and Wilk 2003), and those psychiatrists were not distributed evenly across the population, with rural and remote areas facing particular challenges. Workforce shortages also lead to delays in initial appointments, which increase the likelihood of missed appointments because there is a strong relationship between appointment delay and cancellations or no-shows (Gallucci et al. 2005).

As noted, rural and remote settings are particularly vulnerable to workforce shortages. A recent survey of mental health facilities found that less than half of counties in rural areas have mental health facilities that provide services to children and adolescents (Cummings et al. 2013b), and rural communities have less access to mental health facilities that accept Medicaid (Cummings et al. 2013a). Additionally, because of a variety of factors, including low reimbursement rates compared with those received by other physicians, fewer psychiatrists accept insurance of any type, including private insurance, Medicare, and Medicaid. Furthermore, the number of psychiatrists accepting private insurance and Medicare appears to be declining, not increasing, over time (Bishop et al. 2014).

Societal Stigma and Patient-Level Factors

Even large-scale improvements in insurance coverage and a major increase in the number of mental health professionals would not fully ameliorate the challenges to accessing mental health care. Before engaging with a mental health clinician, individuals with mental illnesses must first recognize the need for treatment or have it recognized by a loved one. They must agree to seek services (unless involuntary treatment is warranted). Although stigma around depression and anxiety disorders may have diminished to some extent in recent decades, the stigma still exists. Evaluation of individuals with untreated depression found that personal stigmatizing attitudes posed an important barrier to seeking care, with study participants reporting lower self-appraisal of symptoms and decreased perceived need for treatment (Schomerus et al. 2012). Dishearteningly, stigma continues to thrive even within the medical profession. A survey of primary care providers and psychiatrists found that physicians believe that their profession holds stigmatizing views of depression and that this attitude relates to reduced help-seeking (Adams et al. 2010). Little change has occurred in the stigma associated with schizophrenia, and even the label of being at risk for psychosis may have a negative impact on an individual's social networks and reduce help-seeking in young adults (Yang et al. 2013). Furthermore, highly publicized mass shootings and other tragedies have been linked to serious mental illnesses in the media and public discourse, which may further increase stigma associated with mental illnesses.

Once a need for services is recognized, individuals (or their representative) must navigate the health care system to request services. This task may involve patients calling a behavioral health access line that is part of their health maintenance organization (HMO) or, as in the example in Massachusetts in the section "Mental Health Workforce Shortages," contacting individual in-network providers or provider groups to request an intake evaluation. Still others must find out which services may have county funding and whether the process is on a first-come, first-served basis involving waiting for an appointment on certain days of the week, a written application process, a scheduled telephone screening interview, or some other variant of the waiting-to-be-seen process. Furthermore, individuals must often coordinate their schedule with the provider's schedule. In some instances in which patients' employers do not post work duty schedules more than a month in advance, scheduling is especially challenging.

Once an appointment is scheduled, many times, an individual must still coordinate transportation to the appointment. Individuals with children must arrange child care options during the appointment. Also, patients must have the financial means to afford any co-pays associated with services. These serial hurdles are repeated for each follow-up appointment. Although these factors have not been clearly quantified, the relative impacts of many personal barriers have been assessed. Using survey data from the National Survey on Drug Use and Health, an estimated 5.2 million adults age 18 or older reported that they had unmet mental health needs and did not receive treatment in the past year for multiple reasons (Figure 10–2). These reasons included, among others, cost (43.7%), belief that the problem could be managed without professional care (32.2%), lack of knowledge with respect to where to find care (20.5%), and not having time (14.6%) (Substance Abuse and Mental Health Services Administration 2012b).

Disparities in Access to Mental Health Care

Although these barriers to access affect the vast majority of Americans, some groups have significantly higher rates of unmet mental health care needs than others. Studies have documented major gaps in the ability of individuals with self-identified need to access services. Insurance coverage is associated with higher rates of treatment for depression but is not associated with higher rates of guideline-concordant care, and the lowest rates of guideline-concordant care are seen among African Americans and Mexican Americans (González et al. 2010). Additionally, racial and ethnic disparities exist in unmet need and access to services, with greater unmet need for mental health disorders, including substance use disorders, in African Americans, Hispanics, American Indians, and Pacific Islanders compared with non-Hispanic whites (Harris et al. 2005; Wells et al. 2001). Furthermore, children (especially children from the aforementioned demographic groups) have high levels of unmet need for various behavioral problems and emotional disturbances (Leaf et al. 1996).

Poor Access to Care as a Social Determinant of Health

The United Nations' *Universal Declaration of Human Rights* states that food, shelter, education, and health care are necessities that governments should provide to their citizens. According to the 2005 Organisation for Economic Co-operation and Development report, 65% of Americans feel that access to health care is a right (Organisation for Economic Co-operation and Development 2005). The World Health Organization defines health care as a *common good* rather than a market commodity (World Health Organization 2008). Even so, striking dispar-

Reasons for not receiving mental health services in the past year among adults age 18 or older with an unmet need for mental health care who did not receive mental health services: 2010

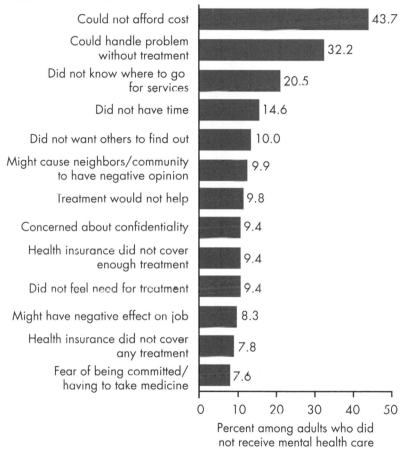

FIGURE 10-2. Results from the 2010 National Survey on Drug Use and Health: Mental Health Findings.

Source. Substance Abuse and Mental Health Services Administration: Results From the 2010 National Survey on Drug Use and Health: Mental Health Findings (NSDUH Series H-42, HHS Publication No. [SMA] 11-4667). Rockville, MD, Substance Abuse and Mental Health Services Administration, 2012.

ities continue to exist in the United States regarding which citizens receive health care and in what manner.

Although the public safety net system in the United States provides some level of care for the uninsured, lack of insurance is a barrier to timely health care and, in turn, results in poorer health, more preventable hospitalizations, and earlier death (Durham et al. 1998; Hadley 2007; Institute of Medicine Committee on the Consequences of Uninsurance 2004; Wilper et al. 2009). That is, those who do not possess health insurance postpone seeking medical attention, resulting in treatable and often preventable conditions developing into serious and/or chronic medical problems. The uninsured poor are two times as likely to delay hospital care as those who are insured, resulting in longer hospital stays and higher rates of death (Weissman et al. 1991). In fact, in a prospective cohort study of adults over 25 years old, the 15-year mortality rate was twice as high among the uninsured (18.4%) compared with those with insurance (9.6%) (Franks et al. 1993). In addition, the uninsured fail to receive necessary preventive screening such as blood pressure monitoring, glaucoma testing, breast exams, and Pap smears (Woolhandler and Himmelstein 1988).

The consequences of poor access to care may be seen in U.S. population measures of health when they are compared with those of other industrialized nations. Female longevity, for example, is 79.4 years in the United States, compared with 81.4 years in Canada and 82.4 years in France (Organisation for Economic Co-operation and Development 2005). Maternal mortality in the United States is approximately 10 deaths per 100,000 live births, whereas Germany, Australia, Italy, Spain, Canada, and Sweden all have rates below 5 per 100,000. Similarly, infant mortality per 1,000 births in the United States is 7.1, compared with rates of 5.7 in Australia, 4.3 in France, and 3.4 in Sweden (Organisation for Economic Co-operation and Development 2005). Of course, these statistics do not imply that these differences are singularly a result of poor access to health care, but access issues are undoubtedly one factor in a multifactorial web of causation. Indeed, in 2000, the World Health Organization ranked the United States thirty-seventh in health care worldwide (The World Health Organization 2000).

Making matters more complex, many of the risk factors and complications associated with the most costly diseases in our society are closely linked to health care access. According to one study, the 10 most costly chronic conditions for American adults are ischemic heart disease, joint disorders such as arthritis, hypertension, chronic back problems, mood disorders, diabetes, cerebrovascular disease, cardiac dysrhythmias, peripheral vascular disorders, and chronic obstructive pulmonary disease (Druss et al. 2002). All of these conditions are treatable, better controlled with early intervention, and considered preventable in one way or another. Therefore, in considering chronic conditions in the United States, the effective prevention and management of these conditions is somewhat dependent on the efficiency, effectiveness, and quality of the health care system. Indeed, survival analyses have confirmed that lack of insurance leads to increased mortality, with an estimated 44,000 excess deaths associated with uninsurance among Americans ages 18–64 in 2005, even after adjusting for education, income, health status, and various health-related risk factors (Wilper et al. 2009).

Poor Access to Care as a Social Determinant of Mental Health

Although it is clear that lack of health insurance and poor access to health care lead to poorer physical health and increased mortality, the association between access to care and mental illnesses is not as direct or well defined. We cannot definitively state that being uninsured or underinsured causes mental illnesses; however, we can convincingly describe worsening of mental health problems associated with poor access to mental health services. Greater attention to the mental health impacts of poor access to health care is warranted.

By examining a natural, randomized experiment that took place in Oregon in which Medicaid expansion in 2008 was limited to lottery drawings, researchers had the ability to observe health outcomes in Oregon residents with Medicaid compared with Oregon residents without health insurance. Although improvements in physical health status were not observed in the conditions measured, substantial improvements in depression were seen among those individuals with Medicaid, including a decreased risk of screening positive for depression (Baicker et al. 2013). That particular study hints at Medicaid coverage as a possible factor in reducing the incidence of depression, perhaps by reducing financial strain and stress associated with being uninsured.

It has been demonstrated that individuals with mental illnesses receive lower-quality medical care (Frayne et al. 2005), resulting in unnecessary hospitalizations that could have been prevented with adequate outpatient care (Mai et al. 2011). Lower-quality care is compounded by comorbidities and medication side effects that result in an accelerating longevity gap, with individuals with mental illnesses dying, on average, up to 25 years earlier than the general population (Parks et al. 2006).

Confronting Poor Access to Health Care in the Clinical Setting

Case Example: Difficulty Accessing Needed Care

Adele Johnson is a 57 year old who presents to her local emergency department with depressed mood, difficulty falling asleep and early morning awakening, decreased energy during the daytime, poor appetite, and suicidal ideation with no plan. The emergency department social worker, Joseph Miller, completes an assessment and determines, on the basis of her risk and protective factors, a moderate level of risk of self-harm or suicide. After discussing Ms. Johnson's case via telephone with the on-call psychiatrist, Dr. Valerie Shaw, the treatment team recommends hospitalization. Ms. Johnson declines this recommendation; she is concerned that she will not be able to afford the loss of income and the possibility of being fired as a result of missing work. In addition, as the primary caregiver for her 3-year-old grandson, Ms. Johnson does not know who would be able to provide childcare if she were to be hospitalized (her grandson is currently with neighbors but only during this emergency department visit).

The level of risk of self-harm does not warrant involuntary psychiatric hospitalization; thus, rapid access to outpatient services is indicated. Indeed, Ms. Johnson states that this was her precise goal in presenting to the emergency department. She reports that she saw her primary care physician approximately 6 weeks ago but did not talk to him about her depressive symptoms because she sensed that he did not have time to talk. She describes one instance of confiding in a trusted coworker about the problems she has been having, and her coworker recommended that she go to a mental health clinic. Ms. Johnson had called a local clinic that the coworker recommended and was told that she would have to wait approximately 3 months for a new patient appointment.

Ms. Johnson has Medicaid coverage, which she anticipates will expire in a few weeks when her youngest child reaches adulthood. She works two part-time jobs that are often difficult to coordinate with each other and with her child care and parenting responsibilities. Although Dr. Shaw considers coming in to the emergency department in order to conduct a complete psychiatric assessment, she is uncomfortable with the prospect of starting an antidepressant medication in the emergency department without proper follow-up being arranged. Furthermore, Ms. Johnson's impending loss of Medicaid may preclude any follow-up for monitoring of side effects and response to treatment. Instead, Mr. Miller, Dr. Shaw, and the emergency medicine physician agree to provide general medication class recommendations, furnish a list of free and sliding-scale primary care or behavioral health clinics and psychotherapy training centers, and encourage the patient to return to the emergency department should she have any further suicidal ideation.

This vignette describes a wholly unsatisfying encounter with a motivated patient who recognizes her mental health needs but cannot access services through the standard channels and thus instead presents to the emergency department. Gaps in health care insurance coverage, coupled with scheduling difficulties and concern regarding necessary follow-up appointments, result in the patient being discharged with limited intervention or resources, with a potential for further delays in accessing care until her illness worsens considerably or until insurance and scheduling allow for the evaluation and treatment she needs. Indeed, these issues are contributors to increasing rates of disability and severity of illness among people with poor access to health care. One wonders what policy and programmatic options might help individuals like Ms. Johnson access needed care.

Policy Approaches to Poor Access to Health Care

Because lack of insurance is a risk factor for poor physical and mental health, policy strategies that promote universal health care coverage could result in improved behavioral health outcomes from a population health perspective. However, political will at present is lacking to move toward developing universal health care coverage. Health insurance coverage is expected to significantly increase under the ACA, making great strides toward improved coverage of uninsured populations in the United States; nonetheless, some individuals will remain uninsured even after full implementation of the ACA (Nardin et al. 2013).

Policies that help promote equity in mental health, substance abuse, and physical health treatment will need to continue to be monitored closely. Significant progress has been made in achieving mental health parity in recent years through the MHPAEA and the ACA. However, in order to ensure that parity in health care coverage is enforced, health care plans will need to be closely monitored, and insurance companies and health care plans that are not in compliance with parity rules will need to be held accountable.

In addition to parity reform, reimbursement reform is needed to address the increasing numbers of psychiatrists and other behavioral health professionals in private practices who do not take insurance. Access problems can stem from the abundance of these cash-only practices, in that individuals who are insured may still be unable to afford quality psychiatric care in the absence of significant disposable income. Along with reimbursement reform, a culture change within the profession is needed to address this growing problem in mental health services access.

Health System Redesign to Promote Access to Mental Health Care

Changes in the fundamental nature of delivery of mental health care in the form of primary care access for individuals with mental illnesses and mental health access in close coordination with primary care (i.e., integrated care approaches) are demonstrating promise for improving access to care. Collaborative care models, which range from colocated care to fully integrated physical and behavioral health services, are effective in increasing access to mental health care by adopting a "no wrong door" approach to behavioral health care. A portion of the population will not seek mental health treatment in mental health clinics or similar settings. Integrated and collaborative care may encourage individuals to access services they would not otherwise seek in settings viewed as less stigmatizing and more acceptable (i.e., primary care settings) (Shim et al. 2011; Snowden and Pingitore 2002). These well-studied models have been shown to be cost-effective as well as clinically efficacious for a wide variety of mental illnesses, especially depression (Gilbody et al. 2006; Thota et al. 2012).

In addition to collaborative care models, programs and initiatives that target quality and performance improvement in treatment often include access to care as a major component. A best practice example is the Henry Ford Health System in Detroit, Michigan, which demonstrates the vast outcome improvements that are possible. Informed by recommendations from the Institute of Medicine report *Crossing the Quality Chasm* (Institute of Medicine Committee on Quality of Health Care in America 2001), the health system developed the Perfect Depression Care initiative, with the primary goal of completely eliminating suicide in the health system. Performance improvement objectives pertained to partnership with patients, clinical care, information flow, and improved access. All patients entering the health system received an initial suicide assessment; those deemed to be at lower risk for suicide were evaluated within 7 days, whereas those deemed to be at high risk of suicide received same-day evaluation services (Coffey 2006). In a short time, the rate of suicide in the patient population dropped by 75%, and by 2010, the health system demonstrated nine consecutive quarters without any suicides (Coffey 2007; Hampton 2010).

Access to Mental Health Services: Policy Approaches at Local, State, and Federal Levels

Despite a relatively high number of mental health professionals per capita, not all communities have access to these providers. Rural communities, neighborhoods that are predominantly African American or Hispanic, and indigenous and tribal communities remain highly underserved (Cummings et al. 2013a). As a result, policy interventions that focus on increasing access to care should consider the unique cultural and societal factors that contribute to poorer access for racial and ethnic minorities and geographically isolated populations. Effective interventions must examine and target these populations in particular in order to better understand what works. Local, state, and federal programs exist for medical student loan forgiveness to encourage individuals to begin their careers in underserved communities, with hopes that clinicians will put down roots in the community and will remain after completion of their requisite service. Similar initiatives focus on training and educating clinicians from underserved and geographically isolated communities because individuals are more likely to return to their home communities on completion of their education and training.

Another promising alternative for increasing access to mental health services is telepsychiatry. The U.S. Department of Veterans Affairs has been highly active in adopting telemedicine for mental health services in areas without mental health professionals, and various other sites have successfully adopted models of telepsychiatry to extend the reach of psychiatric treatment options (McGinty et al. 2006). However, evidence of efficacy and effectiveness in improving mental health outcomes across diverse settings is lacking (García-Lizana and Muñoz-Mayorga 2010). Furthermore, adoption of telepsychiatry as a successful model often requires changes in reimbursement models and considerable systems-level changes to effectively adopt these practices. Still, unique telemedicine programs show potential for increasing access to mental health services, particularly as a method to address disparities in access among rural communities and racial/ethnic minority groups (Shim et al. 2012; Shore et al. 2012)

Promoting Access to High-Quality Health Care: A Role for Everyone

Strategies exist for health care providers to address this social determinant of mental health from a clinical, one-on-one perspective. For example, at the clinician level, mental health professionals can provide evaluation and follow-up appointments outside of normal business hours. At the systems level, psychiatrists and other mental health professionals can advocate for health care system change, whether through the promotion of trials of medical home models, increased collaboration with primary care, or quality improvement and policy initiatives. In their communities, mental health professionals can provide outreach and education, which can prove beneficial both in assisting individuals in recognizing their own early symptoms of mental illnesses and in reducing stigma as a barrier to seeking treatment (Romer and Bock 2008). At local, state, and federal levels, mental health professionals can successfully advocate for their patients through professional organizations and advocacy events. Mental health professionals have a societal responsibility to actively engage in the political discourse to ensure that everyone has the opportunity to access high-quality mental health services.

Key Points

- Barriers to accessing mental health care are multifactorial and far-reaching and occur at the patient, provider, and systems levels.

- Patient-level barriers include lack of insight, self-stigma that comes from societal stigma, challenges navigating the health care system to access care, difficulty with scheduling (e.g., time off from work, child care), lack of transportation, and cost of visit and prescription co-pays.

- Provider-level barriers include lack of availability outside of traditional business hours; wait times of days, weeks, and even months until the next available intake or follow-up appointment; customer service, quality, and performance improvement issues; impediments to rapport and therapeutic alliance; and workforce shortages.

- Systems-level barriers include inequities in mental health coverage, inequities in distribution and availability of the mental health workforce, public stigma, lack of insurance, underinsurance, lack of mental health parity, fragmentation of services, and inequalities within the funding of the public mental health system.

- Poor access to health care leads to poor physical health, poor mental health, increased risk for mental illnesses, increased morbidity, and early death. Individual providers can work within their own clinical settings to begin to address barriers to accessing mental health services. Furthermore, individual providers can join with local, state, and federal organizations to improve access to mental health services.

References

Adams EF, Lee AJ, Pritchard CW, et al: What stops us from healing the healers: a survey of help-seeking behaviour, stigmatisation and depression within the medical profession. Int J Soc Psychiatry 56(4):359–370, 2010 19617278

Ayanian JZ, Weissman JS, Schneider EC, et al: Unmet health needs of uninsured adults in the United States. JAMA 284(16):2061–2069, 2000 11042754

Ayanian JZ, Zaslavsky AM, Weissman JS, et al: Undiagnosed hypertension and hypercholesterolemia among uninsured and insured adults in the Third National Health and Nutrition Examination Survey. Am J Public Health 93(12):2051–2054, 2003 14652333

Baicker K, Taubman SL, Allen HL, et al: The Oregon experiment—effects of Medicaid on clinical outcomes. N Engl J Med 368(18):1713–1722, 2013 23635051

Bishop TF, Press MJ, Keyhani S, et al: Acceptance of insurance by psychiatrists and the implications for access to mental health care. JAMA Psychiatry 71(2):176–181, 2014 24337499

Boyd JW, Linsenmeyer A, Woolhandler S, et al: The crisis in mental health care: a preliminary study of access to psychiatric care in Boston. Ann Emerg Med 58(2):218–219, 2011 21782557

Briesacher BA, Ross-Degnan D, Wagner AK, et al: Out-of-pocket burden of health care spending and the adequacy of the Medicare Part D low-income subsidy. Med Care 48(6):503–509, 2010 20473197

Claxton G, DiJulio B, Finder B, et al: Employer Health Benefits: 2009 Annual Survey. Menlo Park, CA, Kaiser Family Foundation, Health Research and Educational Trust, and National Opinion Research Center, 2009

Coffey CE: Pursuing perfect depression care. Psychiatr Serv 57(10):1524–1526, 2006 17035593

Coffey CE: Building a system of perfect depression care in behavioral health. Jt Comm J Qual Patient Saf 33(4):193–199, 2007 17441556

Corrigan P: How stigma interferes with mental health care. Am Psychol 59(7):614–625, 2004 15491256

Cummings JR, Wen H, Ko M, et al: Geography and the Medicaid mental health care infrastructure: implications for health care reform. JAMA Psychiatry 70(10):1084–1090, 2013a 23965816

Cummings JR, Wen H, Druss BG: Improving access to mental health services for youth in the United States. JAMA 309(6):553–554, 2013b 23403677

Cunningham PJ: Beyond parity: primary care physicians' perspectives on access to mental health care. Health Aff (Millwood) 28(3):w490–w501, 2009 19366722

DeNavas-Walt C, Proctor BD, Smith JC: Income, Poverty, and Health Insurance Coverage in the United States: 2009. Washington, DC, U.S. Government Printing Office, 2010

Druss BG, Marcus SC, Olfson M, et al: The most expensive medical conditions in America. Health Aff (Millwood) 21(4):105–111, 2002 12117121

Durham J, Owen P, Bender B, et al: Self-assessed health status and selected behavioral risk factors among persons with and without health-care coverage—United States, 1994–1995. MMWR Morb Mortal Wkly Rep 47(9):176–180, 1998 9518282

Franks P, Clancy CM, Gold MR: Health insurance and mortality. Evidence from a national cohort. JAMA 270(6):737–741, 1993 8336376

Frayne SM, Halanych JH, Miller DR, et al: Disparities in diabetes care: impact of mental illness. Arch Intern Med 165(22):2631–2638, 2005 16344421

Gallucci G, Swartz W, Hackerman F: Impact of the wait for an initial appointment on the rate of kept appointments at a mental health center. Psychiatr Serv 56(3):344–346, 2005 15746510

García-Lizana F, Muñoz-Mayorga I: What about telepsychiatry? A systematic review. Prim Care Companion J Clin Psychiatry 12(2), pii: PCC.09m00831, doi: 10.4088/PCC.09m0831whi, 2010 20694116

Gilbody S, Bower P, Fletcher J, et al: Collaborative care for depression: a cumulative meta-analysis and review of longer-term outcomes. Arch Intern Med 166(21):2314–2321, 2006 17130383

González HM, Vega WA, Williams DR, et al: Depression care in the United States: too little for too few. Arch Gen Psychiatry 67(1):37–46, 2010 20048221

Greenberg PE, Kessler RC, Birnbaum HG, et al: The economic burden of depression in the United States: how did it change between 1990 and 2000? J Clin Psychiatry 64(12):1465–1475, 2003 14728109

Hadley J: Insurance coverage, medical care use, and short-term health changes following an unintentional injury or the onset of a chronic condition. JAMA 297(10):1073–1084, 2007 17356028

Hampton T: Depression care effort brings dramatic drop in large HMO population's suicide rate. JAMA 303(19):1903–1905, 2010 20483962

Harris KM, Edlund MJ, Larson S: Racial and ethnic differences in the mental health problems and use of mental health care. Med Care 43(8):775–784, 2005 16034291

Hoge MA, Morris JA, Stuart GW, et al: A national action plan for workforce development in behavioral health. Psychiatr Serv 60(7):883–887, 2009 19564217

Institute of Medicine: Care Without Coverage: Too Little, Too Late. Edited by National Academies Press. Washington, DC, National Academy of Sciences, 2002

Institute of Medicine Committee on the Consequences of Uninsurance: Insuring America's Health: Principles and Recommendations. Washington, D.C., National Academies Press, 2004

Institute of Medicine Committee on Quality of Health Care in America: Crossing the Quality Chasm: A New Health System for the 21st Century. Washington, DC, National Academies Press, 2001

Konrad TR, Ellis AR, Thomas KC, et al: County-level estimates of need for mental health professionals in the United States. Psychiatr Serv 60(10):1307–1314, 2009 19797369

Koyanagi C, Siegwarth AW: How Will Health Reform Help People With Mental Illnesses? Washington DC, Bazelon Center for Mental Health Law, 2010

Landerman LR, Burns BJ, Swartz MS, et al: The relationship between insurance coverage and psychiatric disorder in predicting use of mental health services. Am J Psychiatry 151(12):1785–1790, 1994 7977886

Leaf PJ, Alegria M, Cohen P, et al: Mental health service use in the community and schools: results from the four-community Methods for the Epidemiology of Child and Adolescent Mental Disorders Study. J Am Acad Child Adolesc Psychiatry 35(7):889–897, 1996 8768348

Mai Q, Holman CDJ, Sanfilippo FM, et al: The impact of mental illness on potentially preventable hospitalisations: a population-based cohort study. BMC Psychiatry 11:163, 2011 21985082

Mark TL, Levit KR, Vandivort-Warren R, et al: Changes in US spending on mental health and substance abuse treatment, 1986–2005, and implications for policy. Health Aff (Millwood) 30(2):284–292, 2011 21289350

McAlpine DD, Mechanic D: Utilization of specialty mental health care among persons with severe mental illness: the roles of demographics, need, insurance, and risk. Health Serv Res 35(1 Pt 2):277–292, 2000 10778815

McGinty KL, Saeed SA, Simmons SC, et al: Telepsychiatry and e-mental health services: potential for improving access to mental health care. Psychiatr Q 77(4):335–342, 2006 16927161

Mechanic D, McAlpine DD: Mission unfulfilled: potholes on the road to mental health parity. Health Aff (Millwood) 18(5):7–21, 1999 10495588

Millman M: Access to Health Care in America. Washington, DC, National Academies Press, 1993

Nardin R, Zallman L, McCormick D, et al: The uninsured after implementation of the Affordable Care Act: a demographic and geographic analysis. Health Affairs Blog, June 6, 2013. Available at: http://healthaffairs org/blog/2013/06/06/the-uninsured-after-implementation-of-theaffordable-care-act-a-demographic-and-geographic-analysis. Accessed November 12, 2013.

Organisation for Economic Co-operation and Development: OECD Health Data 2005: How Does the United States Compare? Paris, Organisation for Economic Co-operation and Development, 2005. Available at: http://www.oecd.org/dataoecd/15/23/34970246.pdf. Accessed October 20, 2013.

Parks J, Svendsen D, Singer P, et al: Morbidity and Mortality in People With Serious Mental Illness. Alexandria, VA, National Association of State Mental Health Program Directors Medical Directors Council, 2006

Romer D, Bock M: Reducing the stigma of mental illness among adolescents and young adults: the effects of treatment information. J Health Commun 13(8):742–758, 2008 19051111

Schomerus G, Schwahn C, Holzinger A, et al: Evolution of public attitudes about mental illness: a systematic review and meta-analysis. Acta Psychiatr Scand 125(6):440–452, 2012 22242976

Scully JH, Wilk JE: Selected characteristics and data of psychiatrists in the United States, 2001–2002. Acad Psychiatry 27(4):247–251, 2003 14754847

Shim RS, Baltrus P, Ye J, Rust G: Prevalence, treatment, and control of depressive symptoms in the United States: results from the National Health and Nutrition Examination Survey (NHANES), 2005–2008. J Am Board Fam Med 24(1):33–38, 2011 21209342

Shim R, Ye J, Yun K: Treating culturally and linguistically isolated Koreans via telepsychiatry. Psychiatr Serv 63(9): 946, 2012 22949021

Shore JH, Brooks E, Anderson H, et al: Characteristics of telemental health service use by American Indian veterans. Psychiatr Serv 63(2):179–181, 2012 22302338

Smedley BD, Stith AY, Nelson AR: Unequal Treatment: Confronting Racial and Ethnic Disparities in Health Care. Washington, DC, National Academies Press, 2009

Snowden LR, Pingitore D: Frequency and scope of mental health service delivery to African Americans in primary care. Ment Health Serv Res 4(3):123–130, 2002 12385565

Substance Abuse and Mental Health Services Administration: Results From the 2010 National Survey on Drug Use and Health: Mental Health Findings (NSDUH Series H-42, HHS Publication No [SMA] 11-4667). Rockville, MD, Substance Abuse and Mental Health Services Administration, 2012a

Substance Abuse and Mental Health Services Administration: Results From the 2011 National Survey on Drug Use and Health: Mental Health Findings (NSDUH Series H-45, HHS Publication No [SMA] 12-4725). Rockville, MD, Substance Abuse and Mental Health Services Administration, 2012b

Thota AB, Sipe TA, Byard GJ, et al: Collaborative care to improve the management of depressive disorders: a community guide systematic review and meta-analysis. Am J Prev Med 42(5):525–538, 2012 22516495

U.S. Census Bureau: Income, Poverty and Health Insurance Coverage in the United States: 2012. Washington, DC, September 17, 2013. Available at: http://www.census.gov/newsroom/releases/archives/income_wealth/cb13-165.html. Accessed November 13, 2013.

U.S. Department of Health and Human Services: Social determinants of health. HealthyPeople.gov Web site, 2013. Available at: http://healthypeople.gov/2020/topicsobjectives2020/overview.aspx?topicid=39. Accessed November 9, 2013.

Weissman JS, Stern R, Fielding SL, et al: Delayed access to health care: risk factors, reasons, and consequences. Ann Intern Med 114(4):325–331, 1991 1899012

Wells K, Klap R, Koike A, et al: Ethnic disparities in unmet need for alcoholism, drug abuse, and mental health care. Am J Psychiatry 158(12):2027–2032, 2001 11729020

Wilper AP, Woolhandler S, Lasser KE, et al: Health insurance and mortality in US adults. Am J Public Health 99(12):2289–2295, 2009 19762659

Woolhandler S, Himmelstein DU: Reverse targeting of preventive care due to lack of health insurance. JAMA 259(19):2872–2874, 1988 3367454

World Health Organization: The World Health Report 2000: Health Systems: Improving Performance. Geneva, World Health Organization, 2000

World Health Organization: Closing the Gap in a Generation: Health Equity Through Action on the Social Determinants of Health: Commission on Social Determinants of Health Final Report. Geneva, World Health Organization, Commission on Social Determinants of Health, 2008

Yang LH, Anglin DM, Wonpat-Borja AJ, et al: Public stigma associated with psychosis risk syndrome in a college population: implications for peer intervention. Psychiatr Serv 64(3):284–288, 2013 23450386

11

A Call to Action: Addressing the Social Determinants of Mental Health

David Satcher, M.D., Ph.D.
Ruth S. Shim, M.D., M.P.H.

I have been impressed with the urgency of doing. Knowing is not enough; we must apply. Being willing is not enough; we must do.

Leonardo da Vinci, 1452–1519

As detailed throughout this book, the social determinants of mental health are partially responsible for many of the poor behavioral health outcomes and inequities that exist in the United States. However, there is cause for optimism and hope because these social determinants can be altered. Together, our society can create significant change that leads to better mental health and greater well-being for everyone. The first step involves increasing awareness, and this book provides a foundation to expand the knowledge base as it relates to the social determinants of mental health. But "knowing is not enough"; action is required.

Achieving optimal mental health in our society requires considering and then addressing those social determinants that contribute to the "causes of the causes" of poor mental health and mental illnesses. This

The authors acknowledge the helpful feedback and recommendations provided by Michael T. Compton, M.D., M.P.H., Carol Koplan, M.D., Marc W. Manseau, M.D., M.P.H., and Kisha B. Holden, Ph.D., M.S.C.R.

process includes addressing discrimination and social exclusion, adverse early life experiences, poor and unequal education, unemployment and underemployment, poverty and income inequality, food insecurity, housing instability, adverse features of the built environment, poor access to care, and various other determinants that contribute to poor outcomes, including violence and diverse factors that lead to social isolation and poor social support. These social determinants are not an exhaustive list, but they are a place to start. How these determinants are interconnected must also be considered; effective action will require a broad-ranging approach that addresses multiple social determinants of mental health simultaneously.

Our goal is ambitious. It is our vision that every individual, family, and community has an equal opportunity to achieve positive mental health and well-being and that every person has a healthy environment in which to live, grow, work, and interact with society. Although this is a high aspiration, it is achievable. We strongly believe that society can attain this goal and that in order to do so, behavioral health professionals (who encompass mental health professionals and substance use disorder professionals) must play an important role in the process through partnerships and collaborations with diverse stakeholders. The time for action is now. Armed with knowledge, we will lay out a bold plan to move forward by detailing what behavioral health professionals, and indeed everyone, can do to promote mental wellness and address the social determinants of mental health in our patients, families, neighborhoods, and communities.

Key Concepts

Public Health Approach to Mental Health

Poor mental health affects everyone. Given the overall prevalence of mental illnesses, including substance use disorders, and the consequential disability and mortality in this country as well as worldwide, no one is immune to the negative effects of poor mental health and mental illnesses, whether in themselves, in their loved ones, or in society (Mathers et al. 2008). Thus, everyone has a stake in ensuring that active steps are taken to improve mental health in our society. As discussed in *Mental Health: A Report of the Surgeon General* (U.S. Department of Health and Human Services 1999), *Mental Health: Culture, Race, and Ethnicity* (U.S. Department of Health and Human Services 2001), and in Chapter 1, "Overview of the Social Determinants of Mental Health," addressing mental health from a public health, population-based perspective is an effective way to improve mental health and address the social determinants of health. This public health approach requires an emphasis on epidemiology and surveillance, mental illness prevention, mental health promotion, and whole-population mental health.

When considering a public health approach, we must reflect on the McKinlay model, a population health–based model of prevention that describes the importance of "upstream" policy interventions (McKinlay 1979). This model sets the stage for the health impact pyramid (shown in Figure 11-1), which describes health interventions in the context of their impact on overall population health (Frieden 2010). At the top of the pyramid, counseling, education, and clinical interventions are often the types of interventions that happen on an individual or small group level and the types of interventions that behavioral health professionals are most likely to practice with their patients. Interventions that have increasing population impact occur as one progresses down the pyramid and include long-lasting protective interventions and altering individuals' default decisions to healthier ones. Finally, at the base of the pyramid, the most influential public health interventions are actions to address socioeconomic factors. The health impact pyramid emphasizes the role of efforts to address the social determinants of health by implementing effective public health interventions and serves as a guidepost for action.

No Health Without Mental Health

The phrase "no health without mental health," first put forth by the World Health Organization to highlight the importance of including mental health when considering general health, has resonated with audiences, and it is regularly referenced and endorsed by various health organizations worldwide (World Health Organization Regional Office for Europe 2005). The power of this phrase lies in the simplicity of the message: in order to achieve health, any isolation of mental health from health care services, policies, and practices can no longer continue. Health system redesign, including integrated care and collaborative care models, emphasizes the relevance of behavioral health within the framework of general health care.

For action to address the social determinants of mental health to begin, it is vital to underscore the relevance of mental health in the context of physical health. Mental health must be promoted and emphasized as critical to the discussion when considering ways to improve the health of

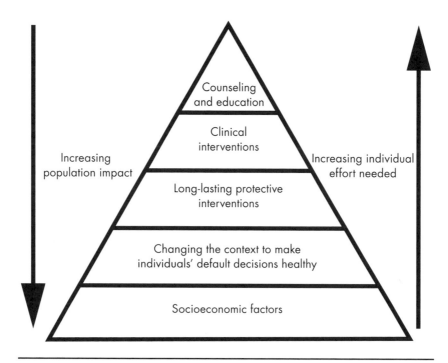

FIGURE 11–1.   Health impact pyramid.

the nation. On a policy level, society must transcend stigma in order to elevate the importance of mental health and the impact of mental illnesses.

Mental Health in All Policies

The concept "all policies are mental health policies" originates from a Health in All Policies (HiAP) approach, which challenges governments and policy makers to consider the impact on health in any policy implementation (Rudolph et al. 2013). Also, the role of multidisciplinary collaborations to improve health in communities is emphasized. Because health issues are complex and interconnected, solutions are also complex and require policy makers to consider multiple factors when making decisions. HiAP also addresses how various governmental sectors (e.g., housing, transportation, education, criminal justice, employment) all have a role in improving the health of the population. Key elements of the HiAP approach include 1) promoting health, equity, and sustainability, 2) supporting intersectorial collaboration, 3) benefiting multiple partners, 4) engaging stakeholders, and 5) creating structural or process change (Rudolph et al. 2013). Examples of using HiAP to improve mental health could involve convening diverse partners (e.g., educators, parents, students, child advocates, policy experts, pediatricians, child psychiatrists and psychologists, community members, funders) to unite for a common goal, such as improving early childhood education programs. Simply opening the lines of communication between various community stakeholders is an important first step. HiAP is discussed in greater detail in Chapter 9, "Adverse Features of the Built Environment."

In a HiAP approach, the natural next step is to consider the impact of policies on mental health. In the "all policies are mental health policies" approach, the principles of HiAP still apply, but governments and policy makers are challenged to consider impacts on mental health of all policy considerations. Health Impact Assessments and Mental Health Impact Assessments, which evaluate the effect of governmental policies and program proposals on community health and mental health, are valuable methodologies for implementing an "all policies are mental health policies" approach (Todman et al. 2012).

Challenges and Barriers to Action

There are several forces that threaten achievement of the goal to provide every American with an equal opportunity for mental well-being. A rhetoric-reality gap exists in taking action on the social determinants of mental health (Larsson 2013). There have been occasions throughout history when the evidence was clearly detailed and the case for action was eloquently made but success in addressing the social determinants of health was not achieved (Irwin and Scali 2005). Therefore, we must consider challenges in advance to effectively make progress. Adopting a strategy that anticipates barriers and focuses on making quick gains is the key to moving forward and taking action.

One major challenge to the effective implementation of strategies to address the social determinants of mental health is the unique policy context and culture of the United States. Our country's political, cultural, and historical background often pits personal responsibility and the freedom to make individual choices against whole-population health and restricting individual choice in the name of the general health of the collective society. When we consider the role of the social determinants, we need to emphasize the relevance of personal responsibility while acknowledging how society and the environment shape the context in which personal choices are made.

Even if society can successfully strike a balance between American individuality and collective health, there are additional barriers in building political will to tackle the social determinants of mental health. The current political environment is characterized by bipartisan divisions, which often presents challenges for enacting any effective policy. Also, prior to convincing lawmakers in Congress, society must build political will and support within the behavioral health field, where neurobiology tends to dominate the conversation about how to prevent and treat mental illnesses and substance use disorders. Additionally, in order to build political will, behavioral health professionals must step outside of their traditional role by developing relationships with lawmakers, collaborating with diverse stakeholders, and increasing their knowledge of public policy and politics.

Another key challenge in addressing the social determinants of mental health is that of competing priorities. Health, in general, is not always the chief priority of local, state, and federal governments. Issues related to the economy, defense, and foreign relations often receive greater attention than health, particularly in moments of crisis. When health is the main focus, mental health must compete for attention with physical health issues, and as a result, mental health care has not always progressed or advanced at the same pace as other health sectors (Mechanic et al. 2013). Adopting an "all policies are mental health policies" approach can hopefully combat some of these challenges. With this perspective, it is easier to consider how seemingly unrelated political issues affect behavioral health and why it is important to include behavioral health when making policy decisions.

Another major challenge in addressing the social determinants of mental health involves the need to reduce stigma associated with mental illnesses, including substance use disorders. Stigma is a complex construct, defined by Erving Goffman as a "deeply discrediting" attribute that can lead to negative stereotypes and discrimination (Goffman 1963). Simply put, it is a corrosive force in the world of mental health evaluation and treatment. On an individual basis, stigma prevents people from seeking behavioral health services in order to avoid being labeled or excluded from social opportunities (Corrigan 2004). Individuals with mental illnesses often receive poorer quality of care for physical health conditions (Sartorius 2007), and psychiatrists often perceive greater difficulty in accessing health care for their patients (Fang and Rizzo 2007). Integrated primary and behavioral health care may help address this stigma and tackle the social determinant of poor access to care.

Even more concerning, stigmatization of mental illnesses has a direct impact on norms and policies. At the population level, societal stigma results in discrimination and can lead to policies and decisions that adversely affect individuals with mental illnesses. Schneider and Ingram (2005) discussed the concept of deservingness in the construction of policies (and ultimately laws) in society. Governance often supports policies that either increase social isolation or ignore vulnerable populations, including those with mental illnesses and substance use disorders. Thus, because stigma exists toward people with mental illnesses, some policies allocate funding to institutions that isolate individuals with mental illnesses, and some limit funding for treatment of mental illnesses and substance use disorders in community settings. These types of policies are illustrated by the "criminalization" of mental illnesses and lack of support for educational, employment, housing, and environmental policies that would improve mental health outcomes. In order to make significant progress in addressing the social determinants of mental health, our society must effectively reduce the stigma associated with mental illnesses and substance use disorders, which will make for more just and fair policy decisions.

How to Take Action

Throughout the United States, there are examples of initiatives and programs, in both the public and private sectors, that are creating a measurable impact on the social determinants of mental health, resulting in improved mental health outcomes for individuals and whole communities. A few examples should be considered in order to highlight how to effectively take action.

Best Practices in Taking Action

The Robert Wood Johnson Foundation has an extensive registry of effective programs and policies that documents the possibilities of what can be accomplished through cross-sector, multilevel collaborations (Arkin et al. 2014). In addition, local, state, and federal government interventions have moved the needle in successfully tackling the social determinants of mental health.

Investing in the mental health and well-being of this country's children is an extremely effective way to affect the social determinants of mental health. Programs that stress early education, especially in the preschool years, have reduced the achievement gap noted in vulnerable populations and, when properly administered, have also demonstrated long-term economic, educational, and mental health benefits into adulthood (Schweinhart et al. 2005). There are many examples of successful preschool interventions. Head Start and the High/Scope Perry Preschool program are the most commonly implemented and studied programs, but Educare, Early Steps to School Success, and the Child-Parent Center Education Program are just a few of the other early educational programs that have demonstrated both immediate and long-term success in children. Evidence has shown that those who participate in the Child-Parent Center Education Program, for example, attain higher levels of education and income, are more likely to have health insurance coverage, and have lower rates of substance abuse and legal problems in adulthood than similar children who did not participate in the program (Reynolds et al. 2011).

Social prescribing, also known as *community referral*, is a method to link patients with nonmedical interventions to address the social determinants of mental health at the individual level (Friedli and Watson 2009). This process can be as basic as prescribing exercise or support groups to patients or as complex as prescribing interventions that address poverty and inequality. Many behavioral health clinicians already engage in social prescribing by referring patients to exercise programs, community supports, or other local resources. However, more extensive types of social prescribing address the underlying social determinants of mental health in the clinical setting. Many effective methods for the practice of social prescribing exist, and Health Leads is one. Doctors can prescribe food, housing, and other basic needs for patients, who in turn give prescriptions to trained advocates (usually college students) who then work with the patient and community programs to provide the "prescribed" resources (Onie 2012).

Because the laws and policies in our country are part of the foundation that creates inequities and the negative social conditions that lead to poor mental health, medical-legal partnerships can address and combat these health-harming policies and enforce and implement health-promoting laws through collaborations with legal staff and health care providers (see Chapter 8, "Poor Housing Quality and Housing Instability," for a more in-depth discussion of medical-legal partnerships). This cross-sector collaboration, first developed in Boston but since replicated and expanded throughout the country, trains health professionals to screen for and identify issues directly affecting the health and mental health of their patients that can be addressed through legal means (Cohen et al. 2010). In Georgia, lawyers, law students, medical students, and pediatricians have partnered to create the Health Law Partnership, which has successfully addressed social determinants of health and mental health for children with asthma and sickle cell disease, as well as their families (McCabe and Kinney 2010; Pettignano et al. 2011).

These examples help us understand what is possible and what can be achieved through innovative collaborations to address the social determinants of mental health. Hopefully, they can inspire behavioral health professionals to do more.

Opportunities to Take Action

If we are bold enough to suggest making recommendations to improve mental health outcomes by taking action on the social determinants of health, then our society must prioritize where and how to take action. As discussed in Chapter 1, the foundational elements that lead to the social determinants of mental health are public policies and social norms, which drive the distribution of opportunity in this country and ultimately lead to health risk behaviors. Therefore, in order to address the social determinants of mental health, we must change public policies and social norms.

Addressing Public Policies

The policies and laws put forth by federal, state, and local governments drive health in a fundamental way. Although not always readily apparent, they directly and indirectly affect mental health and mental illnesses. For example, policies such as redlining, a discriminatory practice of denying services (e.g., loans, mortgages, jobs) to specific groups, led to residential segregation, which in turn led to poor housing conditions and neighborhood dysfunction particularly affecting vulnerable population groups. Although the practice of redlining is technically illegal, the act of redlining is, unfortunately, still covertly practiced today, and vulnerable population groups are still harmed from its effects. The rules, codes, and legislation that pertain to education, employment, food, housing, and discrimination, to name a few, are the foundations that create the social determinants of mental health. In order to effectively take action, behavioral health professionals, working in conjunction with various cross-sector agencies and individuals, need to influence and endorse public policies that promote mental health and well-being.

To change public policies, psychiatrists and other behavioral health professionals must emphasize their role as mental *health* experts, which requires action beyond the walls of the clinic because mental health policies are developed and enacted through relationships with policy makers. In concrete terms, changing policies requires connecting with local, state, and federal representatives. Many elected officials may not have expertise in issues related to mental health and substance use disorders and often respond very positively to constituents who identify themselves and offer expertise and assistance. Such lent support may help elected officials feel more confident in addressing issues related to mental illnesses, including substance use disorders, and can serve to decrease stigma toward behavioral health disorders. This support can be accomplished directly through personal communication or indirectly through various professional organizations, which often have staff who work directly with elected officials.

Addressing Social Norms

Just as powerful as public policies are the social norms that shape our communities. The attitudes, thoughts, beliefs, and values that influence one's worldview can have a substantial impact on the health and wellness of one's community. These opinions and beliefs can be conscious or unconscious thoughts and attitudes about others. They include political ideologies, religious tenets, and views on class, race/ethnicity, gender, and sexual orientation. When society's rules and expectations are focused on caring for and valuing its members (especially those who are most vulnerable), these cultural norms drive institutions and legislators to better address the social determinants of mental health. Those whose attitudes trend more toward ensuring the equality of all people will also help drive positive norms that influence the social determinants of mental health. In contrast, those whose attitudes trend more toward considerations of "us" versus "them" often embrace social norms that favor policies that strengthen the divisions within our country. Therefore, to have the greatest impact on social norms, we need to change people's fundamental beliefs about the value of each person's individual and collective culture and educate people on how to understand and appreciate differences in society. It is important for health professionals to set the social norms of tolerance, acceptance, and celebration of diversity within clinical settings. However, it is just as important to carry that perspective through to interactions with various policy makers and legislators. Also, because social norms are extensively responsible for societal stigma, methods that combat stigma through addressing these norms are necessary to encourage people to value mental health to the same extent as physical health.

Social norms drive the distribution of opportunity in society, and they also affect public policies through the actions of elected officials.

Public policies also affect social norms because it is possible for policies and laws to effectively change societal beliefs about certain issues. For example, in the past, social norms led to a culture that glorified smoking, with half of men and one-third of women smoking regularly in 1964 (U.S. Department of Health and Human Services 2014). Sparked by the release of the first surgeon general's report on smoking and health in 1964 and subsequent reports by every other surgeon general thereafter, laws and policies began to restrict access and exposure to and address the harmful marketing of tobacco products. The dramatic decline in rates of smoking over the past 50 years has demonstrated the effectiveness of policies and laws that drive changes in culture and norms, including the decreased acceptability of smoking (U.S. Department of Health and Human Services 2014).

Addressing the Distribution of Opportunity

All Americans must have the opportunity to acquire safe, stable employment that provides a living wage. Improving employment opportunities through education and skilled labor training is essential. People must be able to live in safe neighborhoods free from violence, disorder, and neglect and in neighborhoods that have collective social capital and are empowered with a political voice to advocate for their needs. Our society must also guarantee that every man, woman, and child has enough healthy, nutritious food and a stable, safe place to live. Americans must demand a society in which neighborhoods support social inclusion and building relationships, rather than isolating people from one another.

Improving access to mental health care and the mental health care system is an important part of ensuring that individuals are able to live healthy lives. This improvement can occur in many ways, including collaborative care, increasing access to insurance and mental health services, and addressing stigma that prevents people from seeking treatment in the first place. As it currently stands, not everyone has the same opportunities to lead a fulfilling, rewarding, healthy life. Simply put, where one is born is a much greater predictor of one's mental health than one's genetic code. Genes matter, but changing the genetic underpinnings of poor health and disease is more difficult than modifying the environment in which someone lives. The underlying social norms and public policies lead to inequalities in the distribution of education, wealth, political voice, and empowerment and lead to a social gradient in which those at the bottom have the least social mobility and the lowest chance to live healthy lives. Those at the top have the greatest chance of continued good health. Of course, this is not to say that individuals at the top of the social ladder do not have mental illnesses and substance use disorders, but if we consider these conditions from a population level, the overall risk is less for the well-to-do compared with those who are more disadvantaged in this country.

What Behavioral Health Professionals Can Do

If policies and norms are the main drivers of the social determinants of mental health, clinicians may doubt the role that they can play in addressing the determinants. However, we submit that sparking political action and intervention is exactly what is needed from behavioral health professionals. It is essential that health professionals take a multifaceted, multilevel approach to addressing the social determinants of mental health. This method of tackling social determinants involves forming close partnerships with multiple stakeholders within society. Building diverse teams that reflect equal representation from various sectors is crucial. Through these partnerships, our society can begin to effectively address the social determinants of mental health.

We challenge behavioral health professionals to take a different view of their patients. In traditional clinical models, individual patients present for treatment, and providers administer some type of clinical intervention. This action is valuable and necessary. Specific action to address the social determinants of mental health through clinical interventions is described in Table 11–1. The suggestions are a starting point to make real change on an individual basis with patients and their family members. Behavioral health professionals can take immediate and direct action to address the social determinants of mental health in practice and clinics. But in adopting a population-based approach, we challenge behavioral health professionals to also consider a new patient: the community. When providers expand their focus to beyond just the individual patient in the clinic to the various people with whom their patients (and they themselves) interact in their everyday lives, the role of the behavioral health clinician in addressing the social determinants of mental health becomes clearer. Furthermore, beyond envisioning the community as the patient, behavioral health professionals can take the additional step of considering the community as an equal partner in addressing the social determinants of mental health. The concern is for

TABLE 11–1. Examples of ways to address the social determinants of mental health in the clinical setting

Social determinant	Action
Discrimination and social exclusion	Use the DSM-5 Cultural Formulation Interview during all diagnostic evaluations[a]
Adverse early life experiences	Screen (using the ACE score calculator) for adverse early life experiences[b]
Poor education	Implement supported education in your practice setting
Unemployment, underemployment, and job insecurity	Implement a supported employment program in your practice setting
Income inequality, poverty, and neighborhood deprivation	Create a local resource list for your practice setting to help support individuals experiencing poverty or financial crisis
Food insecurity	Conduct the one- or two-item food insecurity screening at all initial assessments
Poor housing quality and housing instability	Screen patients with the I-HELP screening tool[c]
Adverse features of the built environment	Educate your clinic and community about mental health impact assessments
Poor access to health care	Consider expanding available appointments in your practice or clinic to outside of traditional work hours (evenings or weekends) 1 or 2 days each week

[a]American Psychiatric Association 2013.
[b]The adverse childhood experiences (ACE) score calculator is available at http://acestudy.org/yahoo_site_admin/assets/docs/ACE_Calculator-English.127143712.pdf. Accessed April 20, 2014.
[c]Information about I-HELP (income, housing, education, legal status, literacy, and personal safety) is available at www.mlpboston.org/about-us/capacity-building. Accessed April 20, 2014.

the mental health and well-being of the entire community, and the interventions become focused on addressing the underlying social and environmental causes that contribute to the expression of mental illnesses within one's patient population. Also, in envisioning the community as their patient and partner, providers can more easily consider their role as leaders of their communities and advocates for community health. As an example, when a mental health professional is treating a patient for posttraumatic stress disorder, the health-damaging effects of his or her neighborhood and community can also be addressed. This might include evaluating and intervening on excessive noise, high rates of violence, limited access to resources, and social isolation among residents.

In the past, behavioral health professionals have not always used their knowledge and influence to accomplish the task of addressing the social determinants of mental health. However, it is essential that they collaborate with various groups, including patients actively receiving treatment, individuals in recovery, public- and private-sector organizations, and on multiple levels within the local, state, and federal spheres of influence. Taking action includes stressing the value and worth of each individual, educating others on the importance of prevention (in clinical practice and in communities), and envisioning the community as a partner in achieving this goal. It involves acting on multiple levels to influence various people and groups. Examples of population-level policy action that can be taken by behavioral health providers are listed in Table 11–2. This list of suggestions is meant to stimulate meaningful conversation about how behavioral health professionals can begin to take policy action to address the underlying determinants of mental health. Table 11–2 gives clear examples of what taking action might look like for each social determinant of mental health discussed in this book. This is by no means an exhaustive list. In fact, it is just the beginning, and we hope that these examples will spark new, innovative plans to address the social determinants of mental health in clinics and communities.

In this chapter we have barely scratched the surface of the work to be done to address the social determinants of mental health and to eliminate health disparities and inequities in opportunities. These great problems of society, including discrimination and social exclusion; adverse early life experiences; poor and unequal education; unemployment, underemployment, and job insecurity; income inequality, poverty, and neighborhood deprivation; food insecurity; poor housing quality and housing instability; adverse features of the built environment; and poor access to health care, all lead (directly and indirectly) to

TABLE 11–2. Examples of policy approaches to address the social determinants of mental health

Social determinant	Action
Discrimination and social exclusion	Read your workplace's antidiscrimination policy and make recommendations to amend any policies that do not adequately protect all groups against discrimination
	Practice and educate others about cultural humility and the awareness that everyone has a unique cultural heritage that should be valued
	Hire people (or encourage management to hire people) who reflect the demographic diversity of your patient population
Adverse early life experiences	Contact your congressional representatives to determine their stance on early childhood education and discuss with them why it is important to support preschool educational programs
	Through your local professional society, partner with other organizations (e.g., pediatrics society, child welfare groups) to increase awareness of the prevalence and consequences of adverse early life experiences
	Volunteer to serve on an advisory board to promote antibullying activities
Poor education	Advocate for the implementation of early childhood education programs for all children in your state
	Partner with your local school system to provide educational enrichment activities to students
	Work with local businesses to create a scholarship fund for students who would not otherwise be able to afford college tuition

TABLE 11-2. Examples of policy approaches to address the social determinants of mental health *(continued)*

Social determinant	Action
Unemployment, underemployment, and job insecurity	Support the development, implementation, or improvement of the JOBS program in your state
	Educate your state representatives on the beneficial mental health effects of providing unemployment insurance benefits to unemployed workers
	Encourage your federal congressional representatives to support a living wage for all workers
Income inequality, poverty, and neighborhood deprivation	Advocate for programs that ameliorate the effects of poverty (e.g., safety net programs)
	Speak about the mental health impacts of budget cuts that would decrease funding for programs that help those living in poverty
	Join an organization in your community that is specifically focused on addressing and alleviating poverty
Food insecurity	Advocate for the protection of federal Supplemental Nutrition Assistance Program benefits
	Join an organization that addresses food insecurity or supports access to nutritious foods
	Visit your local food bank to learn more about the resources it provides in the community and how you can support its work

TABLE 11–2. Examples of policy approaches to address the social determinants of mental health *(continued)*

Social determinant	Action
Poor housing quality and housing instability	Find out if your community has an established medical-legal partnership and become involved if it does or work with national organizations to develop one (using the online toolkit) if it does not[a]
	Encourage your practice to partner with a community health worker who can provide home visits to patients and their families to assess living conditions
	Attend and speak at housing policy meetings taking place within local and state governments
Adverse features of the built environment	Learn how to conduct a mental health impact assessment of a new or proposed policy
	Identify your local city and neighborhood planners and work with them to craft planning policies
	Join the Health in All Policies (HiAP) movement
Poor access to health care	Partner with psychologists and primary care providers to provide integrated care in your clinic
	Talk to your state and federal legislators about supporting policies that increase and expand access to health care
	Work with local coalitions to start a mental health stigma reduction campaign in schools and workplaces

Note. JOBS=Job Opportunities and Basic Skills.
[a]The Medical-Legal Partnership Online Toolkit is available at www.medical-legalpartnership.org/new-medical-legal-partnership-toolkit-available-free-download. Accessed April 20, 2014.

elevated risk for poor mental health, as well as mental illnesses and substance use disorders. An emphasis on prevention is needed to begin to address these problems of social injustice and to begin to take action. Targeted community interventions can have a major impact on individual patients' mental health, but to effect real change, behavioral health professionals must work to develop strong partnerships with diverse stakeholders. Forming partnerships and collaborations in communities across the country in order to begin to tackle the social determinants of mental health could be the greatest impact that behavioral health professionals can make toward this endeavor. As Leonardo da Vinci stated, "Being willing is not enough; we must do." Behavioral health providers cannot be bystanders and must actively work together to ensure the mental health of our neighborhoods, communities, and nation.

Key Points

- To achieve optimal mental health in our society, we must consider and then address those social determinants that contribute to the causes of the causes of mental illnesses.

- To take action to address the social determinants of mental health, it is vital to underscore the relevance of mental health in the context of physical health. Mental health issues must be promoted and emphasized as critical to the discussion when considering ways to improve the health of the nation. On a policy level, we must transcend stigma in order to elevate the importance of mental health and the impact of mental illnesses.

- Public policies, as well as social norms, are the foundations of the social determinants of mental health. Policies and norms affect the distribution of opportunity available for people to achieve good health and live meaningful lives.

- Behavioral health professionals can address the social determinants of mental health in clinical settings, but more progress can be made by influencing policy decisions and attitudes on a population level. Behavioral health professionals must partner with diverse stakeholders to best address the social determinants of mental health.

References

American Psychiatric Association: Diagnostic and Statistical Manual of Mental Disorders, 5th Edition. Arlington, VA, American Psychiatric Association, 2013

Arkin E, Braveman P, Egerter S, et al: Time to Act: Investing in the Health of Our Children and Communities: Recommendations From the Robert Wood Johnson Foundation Commission to Build a Healthier America. Princeton, NJ, Robert Wood Johnson Foundation, 2014. Available at: http://www.rwjf.org/content/dam/farm/reports/reports/2014/rwjf409002. Accessed March 19, 2014.

Cohen E, Fullerton DF, Retkin R, et al: Medical-legal partnership: collaborating with lawyers to identify and address health disparities. J Gen Intern Med 25(Suppl 2):S136–S139, 2010 20352508

Corrigan P: How stigma interferes with mental health care. Am Psychol 59(7):614–625, 2004 15491256

Fang H, Rizzo JA: Do psychiatrists have less access to medical services for their patients? J Ment Health Policy Econ 10(2):63–71, 2007 17603147

Frieden TR: A framework for public health action: the health impact pyramid. Am J Public Health 100(4):590–595, 2010 20167880

Friedli L, Watson S: Social Prescribing for Mental Health: A Guide to Commissioning and Delivery. Leeds, UK, Northern Centre for Mental Health, 2009

Goffman E: Stigma: Notes on the Management of Spoiled Identity. New York, Simon & Schuster, 1963

Irwin A, Scali E: Action on the Social Determinants of Health: Learning From Previous Experiences. Geneva, World Health Organization Secretariat of the Commission on Social Determinants of Health, 2005. Available at: http://www.who.int/social_determinants/resources/action_sd.pdf. Accessed March 10, 2014.

Larsson P: The rhetoric/reality gap in social determinants of mental health. Mental Health Review Journal 18:182–193, 2013

Mathers CD, Fat DM, Boerma JT: The Global Burden of Disease: 2004 Update. Geneva, World Health Organization, 2008

McCabe HA, Kinney ED: Medical legal partnerships: a key strategy for addressing social determinants of health. J Gen Intern Med 25(suppl 2):S200–S201, 2010 20352522

McKinlay JB: Epidemiological and political determinants of social policies regarding the public health. Soc Sci Med 13A(5):541–558, 1979 472783

Mechanic D, McAlpine D, Rochefort D: Mental Health and Social Policy: Beyond Managed Care, 6th Edition. Boston, MA, Pearson, 2013

Onie RD: Creating a new model to help health care providers write prescriptions for health. Health Aff (Millwood) 31(12):2795–2796, 2012 23174811

Pettignano R, Caley SB, Bliss LR: Medical-legal partnership: impact on patients with sickle cell disease. Pediatrics 128(6):e1482–e1488, 2011 22084325

Reynolds AJ, Temple JA, Ou S-R, et al: School-based early childhood education and age-28 well-being: effects by timing, dosage, and subgroups. Science 333(6040):360–364, 2011 21659565

Rudolph L, Caplan J, Ben-Moshe K, et al: Health in All Policies: A Guide for State and Local Governments. Washington, DC, American Public Health Association and Public Health Institute, 2013

Sartorius N: Stigma and mental health. Lancet 370(9590):810–811, 2007 17804064

Schneider AL, Ingram HM: Deserving and Entitled: Social Constructions and Public Policy. Albany, NY, SUNY Press, 2005

Schweinhart L, Montie J, Xiang Z, et al: Lifetime Effects: The High/Scope Perry Preschool Study Through Age 40. Ypsilanti, MI, HighScope Press, 2005

Todman LC, Hricisak LM, Fay JE, et al: Mental health impact assessment: population mental health in Englewood, Chicago, Illinois, USA. Impact Assessment and Project Appraisal 30:116–123, 2012

U.S. Department of Health and Human Services: Mental Health: A Report of the Surgeon General. Rockville, MD, Substance Abuse and Mental Health Services Administration, 1999

U.S. Department of Health and Human Services: Mental Health: Culture, Race, and Ethnicity—A Supplement to Mental Health: A Report of the Surgeon General. Rockville, MD, Substance Abuse and Mental Health Services Administration, 2001

U.S. Department of Health and Human Services: The Health Consequences of Smoking—50 Years of Progress: A Report of the Surgeon General. Atlanta, GA, Centers for Disease Control and Prevention, 2014

World Health Organization Regional Office for Europe: Mental Health: Facing the Challenges, Building Solutions: Report From the WHO European Ministerial Conference. Copenhagen, World Health Organization Regional Office for Europe, 2005

Index

Page numbers printed in **boldface** type refer to tables or figures.